LEARNING RESOURCES CENTRE
Romford College of Nursing, Midwifery & Health Studies

To our wives, Sue and Penny,
who have tolerated and encouraged us
in the writing of this book

Postoperative Pain Control

J.I. ALEXANDER
MB BS, FFARCS, DObst, RCOG
Consultant in Anaesthetics and Pain Relief
Sir Humphry Davy Department of Anaesthetics
The Royal Infirmary
Bristol
and Clinical Lecturer to
the University of Bristol

R.G. HILL
BPharm, PhD
Head, Department of Biology
Parke-Davis Research Unit
Addenbrookes Hospital Site
Cambridge
and Member of Downing College
Cambridge

ROMFORD COLLEGE OF NURSING
& MIDWIFERY LIBRARY
GUBBINS LANE
ROMFORD, ESSEX
RM3 0BE

Blackwell Scientific Publications
OXFORD LONDON EDINBURGH
BOSTON PALO ALTO MELBOURNE

©1987 by
Blackwell Scientific Publications
Editorial offices:
Osney Mead, Oxford OX2 0EL
  (*Orders*: Tel. 0865 240201)
8 John Street, London WC1N 2ES
23 Ainslie Place, Edinburgh EH3
  6AJ
52 Beacon Street, Boston
  Massachusetts 02108, USA
667 Lytton Avenue, Palo Alto
  California 94301, USA
107 Barry Street, Carlton
  Victoria 3053, Australia

All rights reserved. No part of this
publication may be reproduced,
stored in a retrieval system, or
transmitted, in any form or by any
means, electronic, mechanical,
photocopying, recording or otherwise
without the prior permission of the
copyright owner

First published 1987

Set by Setrite Typesetters Ltd
Hong Kong, and printed
and bound in Great
Britain by Billing & Sons Ltd,
Worcester

DISTRIBUTORS

USA
  Year Book Medical Publishers
  35 East Wacker Drive
  Chicago, Illinois 60601
  (*Orders*: Tel. 312 726-9733)

Canada
  The C.V. Mosby Company
  5240 Finch Avenue East,
  Scarborough, Ontario
  (*Orders*: Tel. 416-298-1588)

Australia
  Blackwell Scientific Publications
  (Australia) Pty Ltd
  107 Barry Street
  Carlton, Victoria 3053
  (*Orders*: Tel. (03) 347 0300)

**British Library
Cataloguing in Publication Data**

Alexander, J.I.
  Postoperative pain control.
  1. Pain, Postoperative
  I. Title II. Hill, R.G.
  617'.01   RD98.4

ISBN 0-632-01677-9

Contents

Preface, viii

Acknowledgements, xi

1 **Pain: The Size and Measure of the Problem, 1**
   Definition of pain
   Significance
   Assessment and measurement
   Assessment of analgesic trials

2 **Basic Mechanisms of Pain and Pain Relief, 21**
   Peripheral pathways
   Central pathways
   Chemical messengers of pain

3 **Factors Affecting the Severity of Pain, 32**
   Origin of pain
   Physical factors of the patient
   Psychological factors
   Existing narcotic dependence

4 **Consequences of Postoperative Pain, 46**
   Pulmonary consequences
   Endocrine consequences
   Fluid balance

5 **The Pharmacology of Opioid Analgesics, 56**
   Introduction including endogenous opioids
   Opioid receptors
   Agonists and antagonists
   Alternatives to morphine
   New developments

6 **The Pharmacology of Non-Opioid Analgesics, 82**
   Cyclo-oxygenase inhibitors and related drugs
   Centrally acting cyclo-oxygenase inhibitors
   Nitrous oxide
   Ketamine
   Nefopam

Alpha$_2$ agonists
Flupirtine and tazadolene
Bradykinin antagonists

7 The Pharmacology of Drugs with Secondary Analgesic Properties, 89
Anticonvulsants
Monoamine uptake blockers
Monoamine oxidase inhibitors
Amphetamine and cocaine
Phenothiazines
Benzodiazepines
Transmitter precursors
Other agents

8 The Pharmacology of Local Anaesthetics, 95
The site and mechanism of action
Mechanism of unwanted actions
Methods for prolongation of action
Individual agents
New developments

9 Choices in the Management of Postoperative Pain, 101
Availability of resources
Conditions of the patient and of the pain which affect pain relief
Choices of analgesic drug, technique, timing, and route of administration

10 Regional Anaesthesia and Analgesia, 141
Operative local anaesthesia
Postoperative local anaesthesia: advantages; problems
Choice of local anaesthetic
Nerve blockade techniques to relieve postoperative pain
Reversible neurolysis

11 Spinally Applied Opioids, 175
Administration and spread
Side-effects
Choice of drug and technique

12 Pain Relief for Problem Patients, 185
Neonates and infants
Obesity
Raised intracranial pressure
Day-case surgery
Breast feeding
Convulsive pain
The elderly

13 Pharmacokinetic Considerations, 198
Uptake
Binding
Biotransformation
Excretion
Pharmacokinetic interactions

14 What Next?, 225
Equipment
Manpower and resources
Techniques
Drugs

Appendix I: Drug Interactions, 231

Appendix II: Analgesic Overdose and Its Treatment, 238

Appendix III: Acute and Chronic Pain, 245

Glossary, 247

References, 249

Further Reading, 258

Index, 260

Preface

For more than a decade, the authors, from the departments of pharmacology and anaesthetics in the University of Bristol, have collaborated in the teaching of pain and pain relief to the medical students and to the anaesthetic and surgical Fellowship courses (R.G.H. still gives visiting lectures). The interdepartmental collaboration has had many advantages to all parties, and the integration has led to greater understanding of the mechanisms of pain, and of wider and more rational approaches to its prevention and alleviation. The continuous updating of the information from the clinical, animal, and experimental fields of research has increased the awareness of, and enthusiasm to relieve, postoperative pain. This combined approach would have had little clinical effect without a matching enthusiasm on the part of the nursing staff. Most have not only become more aware of postoperative pain, but have embraced newer effective techniques (such as epidural opioid infusions) with such enthusiasm that they no longer accept the presence of pain in the postoperative patient. They demand or initiate pain relief and/or enquire the reasons for the deficit. Their comments and questions have stimulated much of the study and choice of material for this book. This book is written not only for the anaesthetist, who should initiate pain relief, but also for the surgeons (or physicians) who supervise it, and for those of the medical and nursing staff who administer and monitor it.

It is essentially a handbook, a practical book. We have tried to explain how pain is perceived and modulated by the body and how it can be altered by analgesic techniques and drugs. We wanted to describe how drugs act rather than list their actions so that logical understanding of the actions and interactions of present and future drugs follows naturally. In doing so, we have simplified much of the present knowledge of drug actions and drug movement. To those whose work we have simplified we apologize, and hope they understand the necessity for this. To those who find our approach too simplistic this book was not directed, and we hope they will recommend it to those of their colleagues less expert in pain relief. There are chapters on the mechanism of pain perception and the assessment of its significance and severity. These topics lead not only to an understanding of pain but also to a rational individual approach to pain in each patient. We have sought to explain why the amount of pain is so variable and how we can use that knowledge to choose an appropriate pain-relieving technique or approach within the available resources. We have described drugs other than the conventional opioids, prostaglandin inhibitors, and local anaesthetics, because they may be more effective in relieving pain, and the mechanism of their actions is explained. Also included are drugs which are underutilized or are not yet used in clinical practice, but which, nevertheless, represent an advance in the knowledge or efficacy of pain relief.

Regional anaesthesia and analgesia are emphasized, and where a regional technique is especially relevant to the postoperative period and is one which is not habitually taught it is described in detail. Opioid infusion is a relatively new technique, and the reasons for choosing the drugs and technique are explained. We have included a chapter on difficult problems. These are not the only ones which occur, but are the ones which, in our experience, present most difficulty and whose solutions are not readily to be found in the standard textbooks. There is even a short chapter which presents a very personal view of the requisites for further improvement in this field. We have used small print in the main text to denote passages which are explanatory or of further interest but which can be left unread without altering the sense of the discussion. A book of this size can not be comprehensive either as a reference work or as a source of references. When work has been reviewed or can be found in the books listed for 'Further Reading', or when publications are so notable as to be common knowledge, references may not be given in the text.

However, no handbook would be complete unless it could be used in time of difficulty. We have therefore tabulated, for rapid reference, the medical conditions and drugs which alter, or are altered by, the perception of pain or the method or agents of pain relief. The prediction, recognition and treatment of complications and overdose is set out so that it can be used in times of stress.

We hope sincerely that this 'user's handbook' will be of value to those who feel part of, or who want to be part of, the revolution in pain relief and we hope that they, like us, feel that they are standing on the threshold of a process leading to the elimination of postoperative pain.

J.I. Alexander
R.G. Hill

Acknowledgements

It would be impossible to acknowledge all those who have helped in the gestation of this book. The initiation of the project was the result of discussions with our students and colleagues. Colleagues have given advice and answered questions freely. Our secretaries have typed draft after draft without complaint, and our families and friends have read and corrected them. We would also like to thank Mr Gary James MAA, who has contributed some excellent and amusing drawings.

CHAPTER 1

Pain: The Size and Measure of the Problem

Definition. An unpleasant sensory and emotional experience associated with actual or potential tissue damage or described in terms of such damage (definition of the Taxonomy Committee of the International Association for the Study of Pain).

The value and price of pain

Pain serves as a warning of damage to the individual. Those who are born indifferent to pain, and those who lose their perception of pain, for example due to diabetes, leprosy, syringomyelia, or psychosis, suffer damage, deformity, and loss of affected parts of their bodies.

Pain encourages healing: the sharp pain of a fractured limb is relieved most by immobility, which allows union; the throbbing pain of inflammation is relieved by rest and elevation, which reduces swelling, limits further damage, and encourages resolution.

However, pain is also harmful: the immobility, spasm, and muscular splinting of an injured part causes stiffness, weakness, wasting, and, sometimes, contractures; in the trunk, it inhibits ventilation and causes hypoxaemia; it decreases blood flow and predisposes to deep vein thrombosis and pulmonary emboli; it leads to decubitus ulcers, renal stones, oedema, stress, increased cardiac work, and many other problems.

Development of postoperative pain relief

Postoperatively, pain is usually the result of the operation but may be due to other related or unrelated causes (full bladder, ischaemia, extravasated infusions, etc.), and the diagnosis of the cause of the pain should not be ignored. Once diagnosed, the cause of the pain should be treated, if possible. Any remaining pain should be relieved within the limits of safety to the patient in the postoperative environment. As the dangers and value of postoperative pain relief become more understood, and as the standards of monitoring and care increase, so can these limits be extended.

In 1797, in the battle off Santa Cruz, the right elbow of Admiral Horatio Nelson was shattered by grape-shot. After the battle, the arm was amputated. Rum was the anaesthetic, and postoperatively he was given liberal amounts of opium to dull the pain. Anaesthesia has developed out of all recognition since that time. Postoperative pain relief has developed very little. *The reasons for lack of progress* are many but include certain misconceptions, some of which are still held today:
1 Pain is an inevitable consequence of surgery.
2 It is unpleasant but harmless and always limited in duration.
3 Pain-relieving drugs and procedures carry risks and should be avoided if at all possible.
4 Pain relief obscures the signs of surgical complications and is, therefore, dangerous.
5 Patients are not in pain unless they complain of pain.
6 Postoperative pain is rarely intolerable, and if it can be tolerated by one it can be tolerated by all.

Progress has also been hampered by unsatisfactory methods of measuring pain and by two assumptions:
1 Pain is what the patient says hurts, and, by implication, only the total, subjective pain assessment is valid.
2 All postoperative pain is similar, so that postoperative pain relief following dental, orthopaedic, and visceral operations can properly be compared one with another.

The significance of words for pain

Pain varies not only in severity, but in character and emotional content. Numbers alone cannot indicate the changing experience of pain, and words must be used. Words can relate the kind of pain, and sometimes the mechanism of pain, but they have different shades of meaning to different patients, and they are difficult to use in objective comparisons and statistical tests. Words may indicate:
1 The character of the pain: it may be sharp or dull, throbbing or aching, burning or pulling.
2 The temporal or spatial nature of the pain: it may be constant

or intermittent, continuous, colicky, or convulsive, radiating or shooting.
3 The visceral reflexes and accompanying symptoms: it may be cold, sickening, or numbing.
4 And the emotional effect: terrible, fearful, awful, miserable.

The words used for pain may have unconscious religious or racial associations. From the same Greek root, the word penalty is derived, and pain may indicate or be associated with punishment and guilt. Examples are: 'On pain of death' or 'On pain of forfeit'.
Browning (*Childe Roland*): 'I never saw a brute I hated so, he must be wicked to deserve such pain'.
Pain is used as punishment, usually for children, but even the Christian church in former centuries used pain, even death by torture, as a means of purification from sin. Patients may say 'What have I done to deserve this? and may even be under the unjustified impression that the receipt of analgesics is dependent on good behaviour.

The value of the words is often missed. In general, pain relief is prescribed by one profession and assessed and administered by another. Since the ward nurse has only one or two treatments available for pain of any origin, the diagnosis of the cause, or of a change in the cause, does not materially affect treatment until further referral can be made.

The patient's perspective

For an account of the patient's view of pain, Professor Donald's descriptions of his experiences following two separate cardiac operations are recommended (Marcus *et al.* 1977; *see* Further Reading). He emphasized that the state of mind in which pain is suffered and that in which it is inflicted are most important. The feeling that the medical and nursing staff *care* is comforting, whereas silence, reticence, and callousness make the pain intolerable. Care is demonstrated by preoperative visits by the anaesthetist and theatre nurse, by adequate explanations of the postoperative procedures, and by anticipation and prevention of pain.

Reassurance and care include the explanation that the operation is finished and that such postoperative pain as may occur can and will be treated. A postoperative study in Glasgow (Marcus *et al.* 1977; *see* Further Reading) showed that 48% of patients were unaware that pain relief was readily available. Severe pain is more easily prevented than treated, and pain relief should be *offered* regularly and frequently in the first few postoperative days.

The patient who complains little of pain may:
1 Have a high tolerance of pain.
2 Have a lower rate of metabolism or excretion of analgesics, for reasons discussed in Chapter 13.
3 Be unaware that pain relief is available.
4 Be reticent about admitting to pain.
5 Be unwilling to share his pain experience, or
5 Be unwilling to interrupt the nursing routine to ask for help.

Dalrymple et al. *(1973) showed that the frequency of demand for analgesics was as much a reflection of the introversion–extroversion score as of the amount of nociception experienced.*

The patient who complains more frequently may:
1 Be extrovert enough to share his pain experience with everyone.
2 Have an unrealistic expectation of total pain relief or of unconsciousness.
3 Have anxiety and fear of the consequences of the operation, of death and disfigurement, or have fiscal and domestic worries, or
4 Have need of reassurance and comfort. Fear may be a rational consequence of operation, but it is not socially acceptable.

Frequent demands may result from:
a Inadequate prescribing.
b Rapid metabolism and excretion of the drug.
c Tolerance of or addiction to narcotic analgesics.
d Increasing postoperative pain because of ischaemia, oedema of perineural tissue, full bladder, myocardial ischaemia, and many other causes.

Only the patient knows how much pain there is, what makes it worse, and whether it is tolerable. The ability to cope with, or dissociate from, pain varies from one individual to another, and the use of patient-controlled analgesia systems has shown that some patients require four times as much analgesic medication as others of similar age and weight and following the same operation.

The attendant's view

The reactions elicited by pain-reactive behaviour may vary from sympathy and concern to pity, lack of respect, or annoyance. The ability to tolerate pain is associated with maturity — the ability to defend oneself despite injury. Conversely, the infantile response is one of helplessness and mental retardation. Frequent demands for help or pain relief are time-consuming — the administration of drugs requires two qualified nurses to check the drug, the drug record, the drug stock, and the patient — and detract from the care that can be given to the other patients. This is obvious to the nurses, the other patients, and to the patient himself (who must then reinforce the need for his demands by making further demands).

Nurses and doctors are taught, correctly, about the dangers of analgesic drugs. The respiratory depressant effects of the opioids are emphasized, and these seem to be more memorable than the respiratory depressant effects of thoracoabdominal pain. The result is that less than optimal analgesia is dispensed in most cases, especially when the breathing pattern is abnormal, even when the breathing is rapid and truncated because of pain. Although pain itself is a conscious experience, the reaction to nociception may persist into sleep. Thus, shallow rapid respiration, unnatural immobility, and vasoconstriction, which can give rise to serious complications and which can be relieved by adequate analgesia, may be allowed to persist by those who react only to patient demand.

Memory of pain

This fades quickly. If this were not so, there would be more one-child families and fewer participants in dangerous contact sports. Similarly, patients are willing to enter hospital after one or more operations. If pain is assessed retrospectively, it is scored consistently lower than if assessed at the time of the pain. Conversely, the memory may be enhanced by the spirit of competition: 'the doctors said it was the worst appendix they had ever seen' or 'the nurses said that they had never seen anyone suffer as much as I did'. These statements are usually received with some scepticism, but patients describing untreated pain to visitors and other patients, when pain relief had been consistently offered and refused, increase apprehension in those awaiting surgery.

In most cases, the memory of pain is less than the experience. Unfortunately, this also applies to doctors and nurses, who relate the patient's present pain with their own memory of pain.

Drugs which alter the memory of pain, such as the benzodiazepines, can be used to aid pain relief. It is not true that pain cannot be experienced without the associative memory, and it is also untrue that the benzodiazepines are not respiratory depressants: they can increase inspiratory impedance and the incidence of sleep apnoea. Yet, the reduction of anxiety and anticipation of pain, and the increased muscle relaxation, can reduce the reaction to pain and, therefore, reduce pain itself.

Assessment of pain

Pain is an almost universal experience, yet it remains a most difficult one for one person to describe or relate to another. 'Pain is what the patient says hurts' (H.K. Beecher), but assessing pain by a single global score is no more helpful than describing other emotional sensations, such as the beauty of a painting, in terms of numbers. Yet pain must be assessed if it is to be diagnosed, and if treatments are to be compared and improved. The total feeling of pain must be analysed by division into its component parts:
1 Site.
2 Quality or character.
3 Severity.
4 Associated symptoms.
5 Emotional effect or 'feelings'.

Pain may be assessed directly by the patient or indirectly by an observer, who notices changes in colour, movement, facial expression, and behaviour. It may be judged by tests of the reaction to pain: these reactions may be voluntary (vital capacity, forced expiratory volume) or involuntary (functional residual capacity); they may test pain in the short term (peak flow) or over a longer period (plasma bicarbonate). However, with possibly a few exceptions, they are not specific to pain and are altered by several factors, and by only some types of pain. Pain can also be assessed by comparison, either to previous experiences of pain, to experimentally induced pain in an other part of the body, or to pains which can be relieved by different drugs.

The site of pain must not be assumed to be that of the operation. Pain may arise in other sites: infusion sites, bladder, ischaemic legs, etc. The site of pain is an indication only of the receptive field of the stimulated spinal neurones, and pain may be referred, that is perceived in a site geographically different from that of the organ of nociception, or reflexly tensed muscles may cause pain at a distant site. Examples are the shoulder tip pain caused by gas or acid lying under the diaphragm, and the frontal headache that occurs as a result of cervical root irritation. A change in the site of the pain is usually an indication of a surgical (or anaesthetic) complication and the diagnosis of its cause should be made.

The distribution and radiation of the pain must be assessed. For example, pain that radiates into the groin or leg following herniorrhaphy is suggestive of swelling or irritation of a nerve in the groin. On the other hand, pain that involves a very large segment of the body after a focal operation, especially pain which cannot be localized, is more suggestive of exacerbation by anxiety.

Description of the *character* and *affect* of the pain helps to determine the cause and mechanism of the pain and the most appropriate treatment:
Pulsing, throbbing, beating suggest an inflammatory lesion which may be due to infection or the trauma of the wound.
Sore, tender, tugging, aching are typical of the pain which is felt in the somatic (skin and muscle) structures.
Jumping, flashing, shooting are characteristic of pain of neural tissue — the neuralgias and nerve irritation.
Cold, tight, numb may be used for pain which is associated with nerve compression, or which, like burning and scalding, may be due to involvement of the sympathetic pathways.
Colicky, cramping, crushing are more suggestive of visceral pain.

However, these descriptions are not mutually exclusive: sympathetically mediated pain may occur following injury to the body shell or from stimulation of the viscera, and visceral pain can readily cause reflex spasm of the muscles.

Other words suggest the emotional contribution (fearful, cruel, vicious, torturing), or the reaction to pain (unbearable, nauseating, blinding).

The *timing* of the pain is also useful in deciding treatment. The treatment of sudden, convulsive pain is difficult and, fortunately, is not usually required in the postoperative period. Rhythmical severe abdominal pain may be indicative of incoordinate or excessive peristalsis and can usually be relieved by the opioids, whereas prolonged abdominal cramp may be due to opioid-induced intestinal, ureteric, or biliary spasm. Pain that is occasioned by movement is probably due to musculoskeletal structures, and pain that is relieved by dependence may be due to arterial insufficiency.

Severity of pain

In most cases, the predominant pain is due to the operated wound and organs; the anxiety is treated by reassurance, where possible, and demonstration of care, and the type, amount, frequency, and duration of pain relief are determined by the severity of the pain. Assessments and comparisons of different forms of therapy and different or new analgesics are also made by the severity of the pain.

Subjective measurement of pain severity

1 Simple word scale

The patient is asked to choose the word which most nearly describes the pain. The four words chosen by Beecher as being those least misunderstood were: none, mild, moderate, and severe. The six words in the McGill patient pain index are: none, mild, discomforting, distressing, horrible, and excruciating. The more words chosen, the greater the sensitivity of distinction but the greater the disagreement of the relative value of the words.

2 Visual analogue scale

The patient is asked to mark a horizontal or vertical line, usually 10 cm long, according to the severity of the pain. If the *vertical or horizontal* line is identified by descriptive words (Fig. 1.1), the marks tend to be grouped around the middle of the words. If the words occupy the whole of the scale, less grouping occurs (Fig. 1.2). Better still, if the words are omitted entirely from the length of the scale, it is found that pain of random severity is scored randomly along the whole of the line except at the extremes

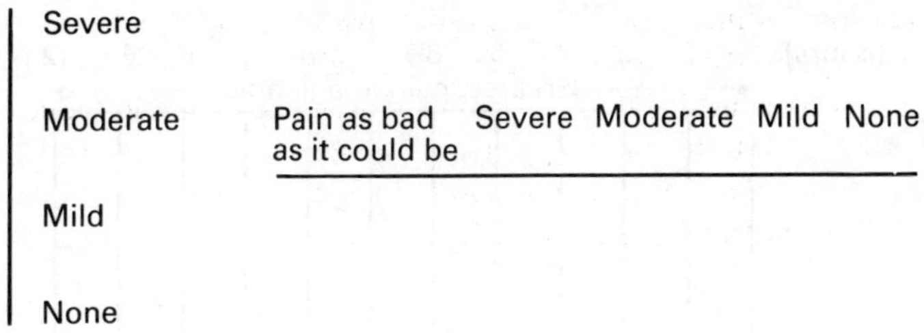

Severe

Moderate   Pain as bad   Severe   Moderate   Mild   None
             as it could be

Mild

None

Fig. 1.1.

(Fig. 1.3). In general, a vertical line is more easily understood than a horizontal one.

A simple refinement is the pain slide rule (Thomas & Griffiths 1982) whereby the patient moves a cursor and the score is read on the reverse side.

The visual analogue scale is simple to operate and easily understood, but reliability is unsatisfactory when the patient is sleepy, fatigued, confused, or uncooperative. It has the further disadvantage that it measures the pain score only at the time of assessment. An attempt to overcome this last difficulty was made by the use of a grid (Fig. 1.4), such that the patient scores the pain at regular intervals and the total pain experienced is calculated from

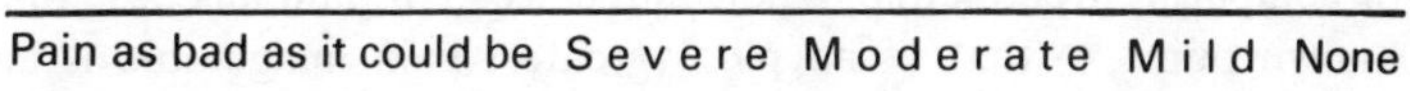

Pain as bad as it could be   S e v e r e   M o d e r a t e   M i l d   None

Fig. 1.2.

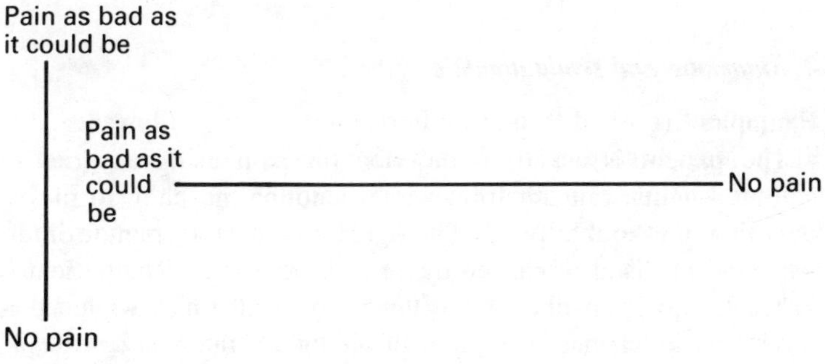

Pain as bad as
it could be

      Pain as
      bad as it
      could ——————————————————— No pain
      be

No pain

Fig. 1.3.

Time
(hours)   1   2   3   4   5   6   7   8   9   10 11 12
◄─────────── Greatest pain imaginable ───────────►

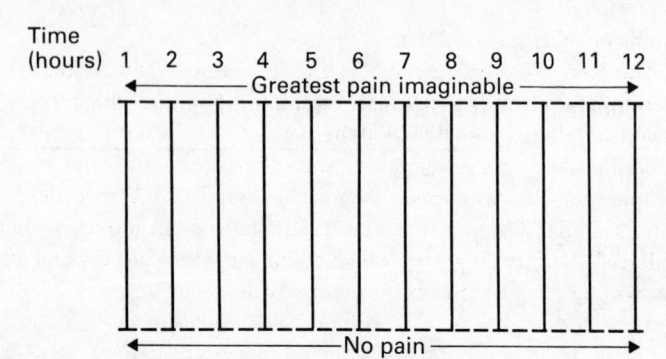

◄─────────────── No pain ───────────────►

Fig. 1.4.

the area under the curve. However, the pain scores tend to be influenced by the previous score so that the curve also measures the degree of pain relief or pain increase.

3 Measure of pain relief

Instead of assessing the level of pain, the patient is asked to assess the proportional decrease of pain following the administration of analgesics or analgesic procedure. This is an equally valid method of comparing treatments. Whereas the score of pain has only one known point — that of no pain (greatest pain imaginable is an abstract and variable term) — that of pain relief has two — no pain relief and complete pain relief.

4 Automatic and semiautomatic systems

Examples are:
a The patient is asked to describe his pain using a series of coloured lights, ranging from white denoting 'no pain' to purple denoting 'intolerable pain'. The lights go out at 15 minute intervals, and this is also marked by an auditory signal. The patient is instructed to keep one of the lights on at all times while he is awake and to change the colour of the light if the pain changes in

intensity (Nayman 1979).

b The King's Pain Recorder. The pain analogue is a 7-cm 30-segment light-emitting diode (LED) display, which can be illuminated progressively from one end by the patient. At preset intervals, the patient's terminal signals ready, and the patient scores the pain by illuminating the display and sends the signal to the recorder.

c In a similar system (Welchew 1982) the patient moves vertical, slide-type variable resistors which change an LED display and alter the position of the pen on a pen-recorder. The severity of pain, nausea, and degree of wakefulness can be recorded.

These systems have the advantage that they eliminate observer bias and yield a continuous recording of the pain. However, they do not measure pain during confusion or sleep and, by repetitively questioning, concentrate the patient's mind on the pain, possibly increasing the perception of it.

5 *Pain scores for children* (and those of limited mental or linguistic ability)

Pain in children may be poorly distinguished from other unpleasant stimuli and situations. Words are replaced by an illustrated scale on which a cursor points variably to a 'happy' or 'unhappy' picture, or the pain can be represented by a pole up which a figure can climb (Fig. 1.5), or by a progressive range of illustrations of facial expressions. (Fig. 1.6).

6 *Pain matching techniques*

An experimental stimulus is applied by the assessor until the pain induced matches the pre-existing pain. Pressure, tourniquet ischaemia, and radiant heat can be used. The inflicted pain can be measured in units of pressure, time, or absorbed energy, and numerical comparisons can be made. However, experimental pain is not entirely comparable: the anxiety associated with death, disability, or disfigurement is (hopefully) absent; the thresholds of pain are different in intact, undamaged tissues from those in tissues which are inflamed; in comparisons of severe pain, some

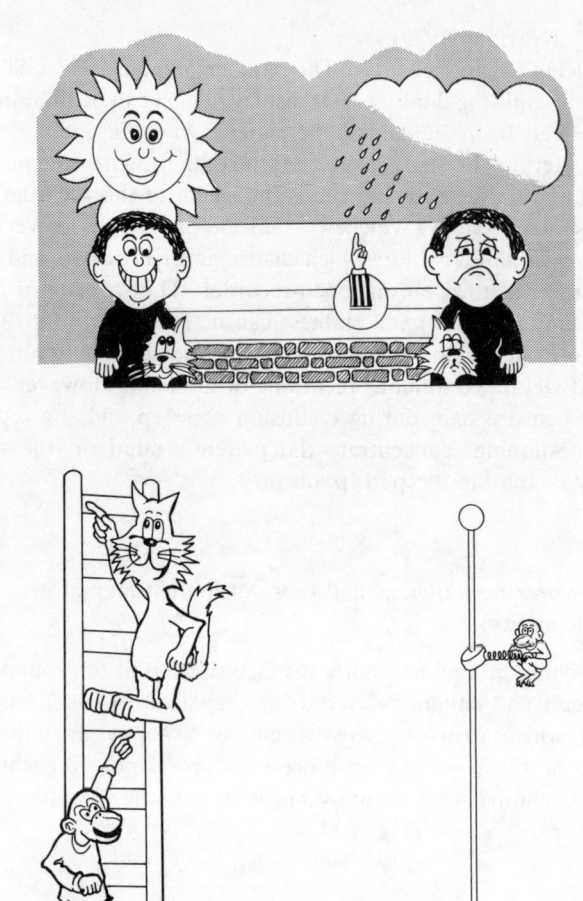

Fig. 1.5. From White & Stow (1985) with permission.

damage of the experimental site is probable, and this will, in itself, alter the pain perception; and the experimental pain may be of different character and be affected differently by analgesic drugs.

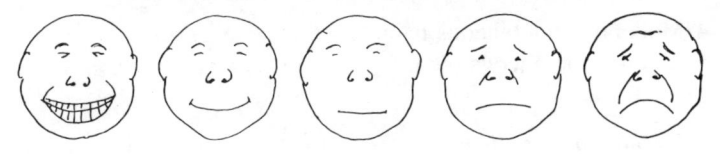

Fig. 1.6. Facial expression analogues of subjective pain.

7 Patient-controlled analgesia

This is used in the treatment of pain and is discussed further in Chapter 9. Briefly, the patient has control of the amount of analgesic administered within certain limits. The amount of analgesic self-administered should be sufficient to produce pain relief or, at least, tolerable discomfort. It is assumed that the amount of drug required to induce this state is proportional to the pain experienced. It has many advantages: the method of assessment achieves the goal of treatment — that of pain relief; it provides a numerical assessment for statistical analysis; and the patient is not subjected to repeated questioning or disturbance. There are disadvantages, too, in this technique as a method of assessment: the rates of distribution and elimination of drugs vary from one patient to another, so that patients need differing amounts of drug to relieve the same pain; drugs with slow onset are inefficient at relieving pain of changing intensity and, without an initial bolus dose, necessitate a period of unrelieved pain; drugs of short duration require frequent demands, such that the patient can become discouraged; pain behaviour in sleep or confusion will not be remedied; and the administration of concomitant drugs influences the assessment.

8 Differential pain scores

Since there are at least two kinds of pain following most operations — dull pain at rest and sharp pain on movement — and since these pains are relieved differentially by opioids and other analgesics, several workers use a word pain scale which scores these pains separately. An example suitable for abdominal surgery is:
0 No pain.
1 Pain only on sudden movement, e.g. coughing.
2 Pain on deep breathing.
3 Mild spontaneous pain.

4 Moderate spontaneous pain.
5 Severe spontaneous pain.

9 McGill pain questionnaire

This seeks to provide a global pain assessment by questioning the site, character and severity of the pain, including the relative severity with regard to time, activity, and previous experience. It is a useful tool in the management of chronic pain, but it is usually too complex for immediate postoperative use.

10 Sensory decision theory

The patient is given pairs of stimuli which differ in intensity in a random fashion. At least one of the pair is painful to the patient. The number of correctly differentiated signals is an index of the sensitivity of the stimulated area (d'), and the rate at which the less painful stimulus is reported to be the greater, or the rate at which the greater stimulus is reported to be the less, is an index of the response criterion (β). The first is a measure of the neurosensory component and the second a measure of the way the sensation is interpreted by the mind. For example, a high proportion of false positives indicates a high expectation of pain, such as might occur in anxiety (Chapman *et al.* 1976).

Objective or indirect measurement of pain severity

Since pain is an interpretation of the perceived sensory stimuli, it is related only indirectly to the nociceptive stimulus, and objective measurement of the perception alone is not possible. However, pain engenders a pain reaction or pain behaviour. If pain is inflicted on any animal, withdrawal of the part, aggressive behaviour, and vocalization are usual. In humans, vocalization may take the form of moaning, groaning, or screaming. Expletives may be used to release aggression. There are facial expressions which one learns to associate with pain. There are autonomic and biochemical changes. Further painful stimuli are avoided. These may include deep or normal breathing.

These changes can be measured by an observer and used in

comparisons with other patients who have similar pains from similar sites.

11 Respiratory changes

(a) Blood gases and rate of ventilation

Although there are changes in respiratory drive and in lung capacities during all kinds of anaesthesia and surgery, the greatest postoperative reduction of lung volumes, capacities, and ventilatory function follows thoracic and upper abdominal surgery. Movement of the injured part is 'painful' and is reduced even when the patient is asleep. The inspiration is truncated, i.e. it is terminated early and abruptly and is followed by a pause before expiration. The ventilation is shallow and there is a tendency for the tension of carbon dioxide to rise and for that of oxygen to fall. Both factors increase the ventilatory rate. This has a greater effect on the carbon dioxide tension than on the oxygen tension, and the net result is lowered tensions of both carbon dioxide *and* oxygen.

(b) Lung volumes and capacities

Not only is breathing, especially deep breathing, painful but, because of the reasons which will be outlined in Chapter 3, the lung volumes and capacities are reduced in the presence of abdominal wall pain. The rate of expiration (or inspiration) is reduced, and so is the amount of expiration. These can be measured readily by the bedside by a peak flow meter and a spirometer respectively. Both are very dependent on the motivation and effort of the patient.

The functional residual capacity (FRC), i.e. the volume of the lung at the end of passive expiration, is also reduced by abdominal wall spasm and is independent of voluntary effort. This can be measured by the helium or nitrogen dilution technique. Because the FRC falls because of forces outside the lung, and because airways close at a more constant lung volume, after thoracic and abdominal surgery airways close earlier in expiration (Alexander *et al.* 1973). The point of airway closure can be measured by a single-breath analysis and the 'closing volume' estimated.

12 Biochemical tests

Acute pain is accompanied by anxiety and other autonomic and hormonal disturbances. It causes increases in the levels of adrenaline, noradrenaline, and serotonin, but these increases are also associated with other forms of stress, including that of venepuncture. Fell *et al.* (1982) have shown no correlation between plasma catecholamine concentrations and linear analogue scores of pain in the postoperative period. Plasma levels of cortisol and antidiuretic hormone rise in response to pain, but also in response to other forms of stress, such as surgery.

The levels of endogenous opioids in the brain, blood, and CSF are altered by pain. The level of beta-endorphin-like immunoreactivity (β-ELI) in CSF is lower in postoperative patients than in controls, and a low *preoperative* plasma β-ELI predicts a large requirement of postoperative analgesia (Cohen *et al.* 1982). However, Fletcher (1985) showed that in labour, despite a rising β-ELI level, there was no correlation of pain tolerance with β-ELI in individual patients.

13 Electroencephalography

A brief painful stimulus produces a detectable evoked potential in a simple two-lead occipitofrontal electroencephalograph. The height of the cortical deflection is linearly related to the intensity of the stimulus (Chapman *et al.* 1979). Nitrous oxide, transcutaneous electrical stimulation, and acupuncture can reduce the height of this deflection. The applicability of this technique to monitoring of the pain experience has yet to be established.

Assessment of analgesic trials

There are many trials of new analgesic drugs and methods, and the majority are shown to be as good or better than the standard or control methods and drugs. Despite the advances in recent years, most of these new drugs and techniques are not adopted and fall into disuse. Why are not more improvements adopted? Are the innovations too expensive in terms of finance, time, or personnel, or are, perhaps, the original conclusions misguided or overenthusiastic?

Overenthusiastic conclusions

Following a long, carefully conducted study, there is a natural desire to make a positive statement, but the form of words used may not be justified. For example, the phrase: 'there was found to be no difference between A and B' is used when the authors merely failed to find a difference. Indeed, in many cases, the design of trial, the choice of methods, the number of subjects chosen for study, and the variation within the general population make it unlikely that a difference, or lack of it, can be demonstrated.

Many readers read only the summary of articles. Explanations of results which are suppositions and untested by previous or subsequent experiment should be confined to the discussion section and not transposed to the summary.

Design of study

Pain is not a single entity and the *choice of operation* affects the efficacy of the postoperative medication. Low doses of opioids affect the unpleasant nature of pain, whereas the non-steroidal anti-inflammatory analgesics (NSAIDs) act principally by restoring the pain threshold toward normal and are most effective for inflammatory pain. If the pain following dental surgery, episiotomy, and minor orthopaedic operations is chosen for study, NSAIDs may be as effective as low doses of opioids. This does not apply for all forms of postoperative pain.

NSAIDs and local anaesthetics have less effect than the opioids on the anxiety or fear of the consequences of surgery and the exaggeration of pain and discomfort they cause. The additional attention to, and monitoring of, the patient during analgesic trials increase the reassurance and reduce the differences in pain complaint following these drugs.

The *individual variation* of response to and elimination of drugs is very large, and these factors are considered in Chapters 3 and 13. The individual variation varies also with the drug, e.g. patient variability is greater for pethidine than for morphine.

The *timing of the drugs* affects the result. Postoperative pain tends to diminish with time. If drugs are tested consecutively, the second will appear to be more effective than the first, especially if there is a residual effect from the first drug. Test and control drugs should precede and follow each other randomly or in matched pairs.

The apparent effect of a drug depends upon not only the absolute efficacy and potency of the drug, but also the relationship of the time of peak onset and the duration of effect to *the time of testing*. For example, when pentazocine was compared to morphine, its potency was exaggerated when analgesia was tested after 20 minutes and diminished when tested after four hours.

Placebo effect

Any procedure which the patient undergoes with the intention of relieving pain will relieve pain in a proportion (approximately one-third) of patients. The greater the confidence expressed by the administrator, the greater the faith of the patient, and the more dramatic the procedure, the greater will be this proportion. The placebo effect is probably mediated by the endogenous opioid systems and, thus, may be blocked by naloxone. It is of considerable benefit in normal clinical practice, providing analgesia with few, if any, side-effects, but the placebo effect should be the same in the groups under test or the effect itself must be estimated. The form of administration, monitoring, and equipment must be the same in each group, and this may necessitate the use of dummy tablets or injections. When the drug is administered in an invasive way, e.g. intrathecally, this may involve an additional risk to the patient with no concomitant benefit. The patient volunteer must be aware of this. The use of dummy medication alone is considered inadequate and unethical for postoperative pain, so that the placebo effect cannot be measured directly. Analgesic trials themselves have a placebo effect, and retrospective comparisons of drugs or methods can be misleading.

Analysis of results

The difficulties of pain measurement have already been mentioned. The numbers derived from pain scores of subjective assessments are not related to each other in an arithmetical sense but are used instead of an infinite number of words with variable meaning.

A pain score of 6 cannot be said to represent twice as much pain as a pain score of 3, and the score numbers should be treated as a number of ranks or steps. It follows that mean pain scores or standard deviations are without meaning, yet they are frequently used to demonstrate a statistical significance or difference. Nonparametric tests should be used for these data. Other forms of data, such as amounts or frequency of medication, are expressed in real numbers and are more suitable for parametric analysis.

Despite the difficulties of demonstrating differences in pain relief, whether or not they are present, there is no doubt that some improvements can be made.

The cost of analgesic modification

As in other branches of medicine, the cost of new drugs is almost always greater than that of the older counterparts. Yet the cost of the drug alone does not appear to be the main deciding factor in analgesia. Pentazocine made a considerable penetration into postoperative analgesia despite being 10 times the cost of papaveretum. The main cost of improved analgesia is in equipment and in medical and nursing time. Infusion pumps, transcutaneous nerve stimulators, monitoring equipment, and patient-controlled analgesia devices are all expensive in the quantity and availability required. The time spent on the repeated administration and constant monitoring required for optimal analgesia is not usually available with the present staffing levels in the U.K. Although pain itself is a potent cause of morbidity, the safety and cost of the method of analgesia is at least as important for its adoption as is its efficacy.

Summary

Pain is an unpleasant perception of harmful stimuli and is modified by associations of that perception. Pain promotes the avoidance of further damage. However, the reaction to pain may also be harmful, and postoperative pain relief reduces the prevalence of suffering and postoperative complications. Improvement of methods of pain relief is hampered partly by the inadequacy of the present means of assessment of pain. Pain varies in character, site, severity, timing, and affect. It can be assessed either by the subjective judgement of the sufferer or by the subjective estimate or objective measurement of the sufferer's reaction to the pain. Progress can be made only by increasing our knowledge of pain and by controlled trials of pain-relieving drugs and techniques, properly designed and accurately reported.

CHAPTER 2
Basic Mechanisms of Pain and Pain Relief

Those fibres which carry sensory messages from the tissues of the body to the central nervous system are similar in that they are all pseudounipolar neurones with their cell bodies in the dorsal root ganglia close to the spinal cord (Fig. 2.1). They differ, however, in that they occur in a variety of sizes, and only the smaller sensory fibres are thought to have an important role in pain perception. The smallest and the most numerous fibres are the C or unmyelinated type, and the others that are generally considered relevant to pain perception are the Aδ or small myelinated type. For electronic reasons the small fibres conduct impulses very slowly (at between 0.1 and 4 m/s). As motor reactions to painful stimuli can occur very rapidly, this must sometimes involve the larger sensory fibres, i.e. Aα and Aβ types, that we do not normally associate with pain perception. It is also evident that in the presence of nerve injury there may be increased involvement of larger myelinated fibres in pain perception as well as in physical reactions to pain.

The most relevant recent studies on sensory nerve physiology are those conducted in human volunteers by Torebjork and his colleagues in Sweden (Hallin *et al.* 1982). A combination of electrophysiological and psychophysical techniques has been used to

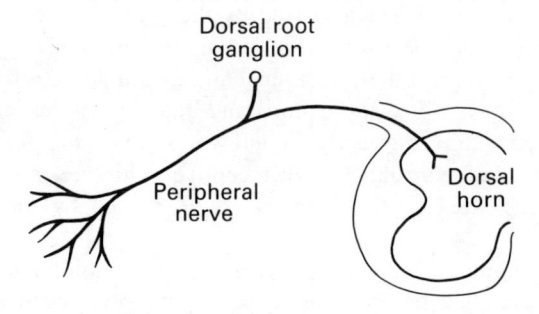

Fig. 2.1. Reproduced with permission from Hill R.G. (1986) *Science Progress* **70**, 95–107.

relate the activity of sensory fibres in peripheral nerves to the experience of pain or other sensation evoked by various types of stimulation. In general, activity in C fibres shows the best correlation with the subject's reporting of painful sensation, and those Aδ fibres that respond to noxious stimuli have a somewhat higher threshold than the psychophysical pain threshold.

The method used involves insertion of a tungsten microelectrode into a peripheral nerve bundle of a conscious subject whilst monitoring the evoked electrical activity in response to physical or electrical stimuli. It is possible to obtain recordings from a small number of fibres such that the activity of a single fibre can be discriminated. When a fibre that can be characterized as a C fibre on the basis of response to noxious stimuli and conduction velocity is found, the experimental arrangement is reversed such that the recording microelectrode is used as a stimulating electrode instead, and the subject is asked to report his subjective experience. The first and frequently the only sensation reported is one of pain.

It is only fair to point out that there are many technical difficulties in explaining these experiments (e.g. how do electrodes that are many times larger than the nerve fibre being stimulated or recorded from manage to select a few from bundles containing many?) and that not all pain experts agree on their usefulness. However the observations made show a striking correspondence with deductions based on other experimental evidence, particularly from well-controlled studies on animals.

Single shocks do not cause a painful sensation as readily as repetitive stimulation, and the higher the frequency of the stimulus train the sooner pain is reported by the subject. The conclusion drawn from these studies is that coding of pain intensity (particularly in response to thermal injury) and threshold detection is the function of C fibre nociceptors and that Aδ fibres are more concerned with pain localization and with sensitization phenomena. Both types of fibre have small receptive fields, i.e. a comparatively small area of tissue seems to be served by the sensory endings.

The other functions of nociceptive sensory afferents are perhaps best considered in terms of the relative conduction velocities of the fibre types involved. When a part of the body is injured impulses travelling in Aδ fibres are the first to reach the central nervous system, and the sensation of sharp or first pain is experienced. Following this, after a perceptible interval, impulses travelling in C fibres also arrive and lead to the experience of dull or second pain. The body's reflex responses to these two sets of information are quite different, and whereas input from Aδ fibre afferents produces protective withdrawal (flexion) reflexes, that from C fibres tends to produce immobility (guarding) (*see* Table 2.1).

It has been suggested that some pathological pain states might be due to an imbalance in the relative numbers of C and A fibres in sensory nerves, and the pain of post-herpetic neuralgia has been cited as an example of this. Recent anatomical and physiological studies have questioned this conclusion however, and it is advisable to regard the matter as open to doubt.

The dorsal horn of the spinal cord

Most sensory axons enter the spinal cord by way of the dorsal root (Fig. 2.1), but some of the smaller fibres are now known to enter by way of the ventral root. Once within the grey matter of the spinal cord, sensory information is relayed to higher centres of the nervous system by way of synaptic contacts made with a variety of relay neurones situated within the dorsal horn. This passage of information upwards is obviously the reason for the conscious

Table 2.1. Summary of differences between first and second pain. From Bowsher (1981) with permission.

	First pain (fast)	Second pain (slow)
Adequate stimulus	Pinprick, heat	Tissue damage
Sensory units	Aδ mechanical and mechanical–thermal nociceptors	C polymodal nociceptors
Distribution	Body surface, including mouth and anus	Most tissues, superficial and deep
Reflex reaction	Phasic muscle contraction — withdrawal	Tonic muscle contraction — spasm, guarding, rigidity
Effect of morphine (therapeutic dose)	None or very little	Suppression

perception of pain, but it is also important to remember that part of the response to a painful stimulus is expressed by way of a local spinal reflex. As mentioned earlier, activity in the larger myelinated fibres leads to an immediate avoidance or flexion reflex, such as the abrupt removal of a limb from the vicinity of a damaging stimulus, whereas the reflex response to C fibre activation is usually immobility or guarding (and this latter effect may also involve descending influences from higher centres). This spinal part of the response to pain does not entirely depend on the brain, and it can be convincingly demonstrated in patients with complete spinal transection that a vigorous withdrawal reflex occurs in response to noxious stimulation of a limb below the level of transection, even though the patient does not experience any sensation as a result of the stimulus.

Returning to those neurones that are responsible for onward transmission of the pain message, these can be broadly classified into two categories (Fig.2.2). Firstly, there are small neurones localized relatively superficially (within lamina II, the substantia gelatinosa) which predominantly receive input from small-diameter C fibres. Although some of these small neurones may have axons that ascend to higher centres, most appear to synapse within the segment of entry, or at most one above or below, and appear to be involved with the spatial and modality convergence of information onto neurones situated in the deeper layers of the dorsal horn. The second category, comprising the larger sensory neurones, can be further subdivided into two main types.

a Those situated in lamina I, the most superficial part of the dorsal horn grey matter, receive inputs from a small number of C or Aδ fibres only. They consequently have small sensory receptive fields, corresponding to those of the fibres that feed them, and may have a role in localizing the part of the body where pain is being generated. These neurones have axons that cross over into the anterolateral tract on the opposite side of the spinal cord and ascend therein to the brainstem and thalamus.

b Large sensory neurones found within the deeper part of the dorsal horn (typically lamina V) have rather different properties to the superficial neurones described above. These neurones can typically be excited by noxious stimuli applied to a comparatively

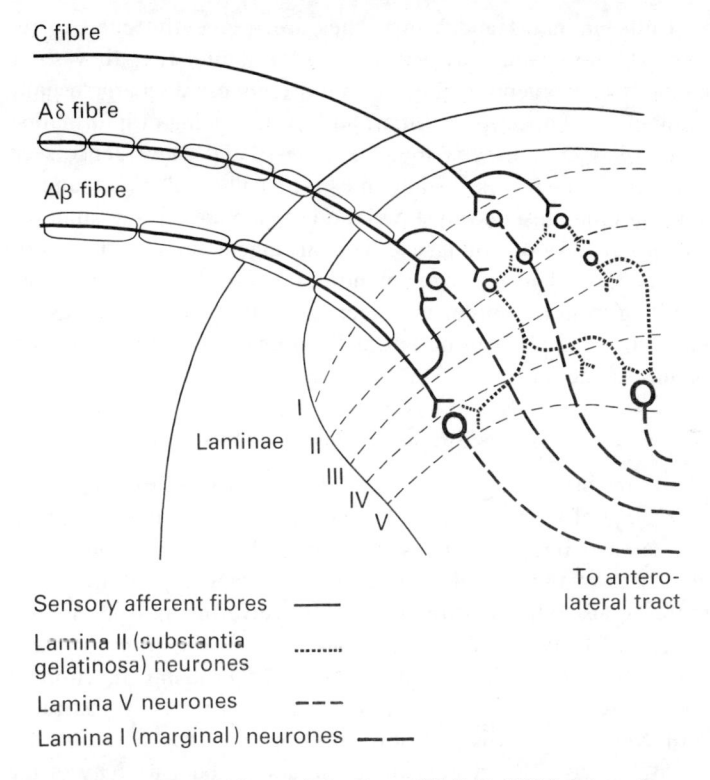

Fig. 2.2. Reproduced with permission from Hill R.G. (1986) *Science Progress* **70**, 95–107.

wide area of the body surface and therefore must receive inputs from a large number of sensory nociceptive peripheral nerve fibres (probably relayed by way of some of the small neurones within the substantia gelatinosa). This lack of spatial discrimination suggests that this type of neurone may more adequately serve to code pain intensity rather than its location. In common with the lamina I neurones the axons of those in lamina V cross the spinal cord and ascend in the contralateral anterolateral tract to the brainstem, and in some cases to the thalamus. Recent evidence suggests that, whereas the above arrangement may well be correct for skin afferents, there may be a different pattern for visceral and some muscle afferents in which small fibres pass direct to lamina V neurones.

Both laminae I and V neurones are frequently found to respond to non-painful as well as painful stimuli (i.e. they show modality convergence), although a more intense discharge usually results from a nociceptive input, and so the coding of information sent to higher centres is complex. The spatial convergence seen in lamina V neurones is sometimes rather illogical. For example, neurones may respond to stimulation of skin and also to stimulation of gut, bladder or testes. This arrangement does, however, help us to explain the phenomenon of referred pain, where pain resulting from a disorder in a deep visceral structure, such as the heart for example, can be felt as apparent pain in the superficial tissues of the left arm.

The brainstem and thalamus

The fibres originating in the spinal dorsal horn and running in the anterolateral tracts first synapse with neurones in the brainstem. This area is one of complex function and complex connectivity. Neurones in the reticular formation and central grey areas (for more details refer to Brodal [1981]) receive inputs from anterolateral tract fibres and then send their own axons both upwards and downwards. The upward projections probably function to convey pain intensity information to higher centres, whilst those projecting downwards probably contribute to the operation of a negative feedback circuit that can modulate the sensitivity of the central nervous system to a painful stimulus and also have a role in the inhibitory control of nociceptive motor reflexes (*see later* for consideration of the role of neurotransmitters in this process).

Some anterolateral tract fibres, notably those originating from neurones in lamina I of the spinal cord, project to the thalamus directly without intermediate synapses (the spinothalamic tract), and this input is probably the principal source of information on the location of pain. A large part of the input to the thalamus comes from the axons of neurones in the brainstem that receive input from the anterolateral tract as described above. It is noteworthy that an imbalance in the relative activity of different thalamic nuclei (usually caused by a pathological lesion) leads to the intractable pain of the thalamic syndrome.

The cerebral cortex

There is still a certain amount of confusion about the role of the cortex in pain perception. It undoubtedly does have a function, as pain quite definitely impinges on consciousness and consciousness is an exclusively cortical phenomenon. It is probably true to say, however, that there is not a cortical 'pain centre' as such, but that the consequences of painful input are exerted in a diffuse way. It has been suggested that pain information reaches the limbic system (often called the seat of the emotions) by way of the cortex, and thus the degree of 'suffering' may be under direct cortical control. The brainstem nuclei involved in descending feedback control also receive cortical inputs, and thus a proportion of the descending inhibitory control of spinal cord and brainstem nociceptive neurones may originate in cortical processing. It is important to remember that pain can often (but not always) be well localized by the patient, and this presumably occurs at a cortical level.

Chemical messengers and pain

An underlying characteristic of the whole pain perception process is the involvement of chemical messengers. The initial damaging trauma or disease state that initiates pain probably does so by release of pain-producing substances (or algogens) within the peripheral tissues and viscera. These algogens then stimulate undifferentiated nerve fibre terminals leading to action potential generation in $A\delta$ and C fibres. When these impulses arrive via the sensory nerve fibres and sensory roots in the spinal cord the message is relayed to dorsal horn interneurones by means of a second set of chemical messengers or neurotransmitters released from the terminals of the afferent sensory fibres. The signal is then carried up to higher centres (ultimately the cerebral cortex) by a chain of neurones all releasing their characteristic chemical messages.

The modulation of pain perception by segmental and descending inhibitory processes also involves neurotransmitters, only this time acting to inhibit synaptic transmission. A knowledge of the principles of neurotransmission and of neurotransmitter substances is therefore important to an undertstanding of the physiology of pain perception. Although less immediately obvious, it is also important if one is to have an adequate conception of the mode of action of pain-relieving (or analgesic) drugs.

How tissue damage and inflammation cause pain

Although it is possible for nerve impulses to be generated as a result of physical movement of nerve fibres (perhaps as a result of changes in membrane capacitance) it is likely that the prime factor underlying the production of afferent nerve activity by injury is that tissue damage releases pain-producing chemicals (algogens). These algogens then interact with receptor sites on afferent nerve terminals producing an increase in ionic conductance that then leads to action potential generation. Algogens are a diverse group of chemicals ranging from K^+ ions through acetylcholine, histamine, and 5-hydroxytryptamine to peptides such as bradykinin. Most of these substances can easily be demonstrated to cause pain in man if injected percutaneously or if applied to an experimental blister base. Some interaction between algogens occurs, and it is likely that the pathophysiological response which leads to the production of the sensation we call pain is attributable to a number of substances acting in concert. Prostanoids are substances well known to be released into inflamed tissues, and they can act to sensitize nociceptor terminals to algogens, although prostanoids themselves, when experimentally administered, do not appear to be capable of evoking pain directly.

The pseudounipolar fibres that are normally thought of as nociceptive primary afferents can release chemical mediators at their peripheral as well as at their central ends. It is possible that such release contributes to nociceptive responses. Most of the substances so far isolated from sensory C fibres are small peptides such as substance P and somatostatin (which will be discussed later). Although the study of the peripheral action of small peptides is incomplete, experiments with pure synthetic substance P suggest that their presence in the tissues does not by itself cause pain. It is more likely that the importance of substances such as substance P is in increasing local blood flow, although the precise effect of such an action on pain remains to be elucidated. Synthetic substance P antagonist peptides will block the peripheral vasodilation caused by exogenous substance P or by antidromic stimulation of a peripheral nerve. It has also been observed that rats with a chronic inflammatory disorder (polyarthritis) have elevated levels of substance P in their peripheral nerves. It is possible that many peptides other than substance P can be released from the peripheral ends of nerve fibres that contain them, and elucidation of the precise role of these substances may have great significance for our understanding of pain perception.

Another group of small fibres known to have an association with pain are the sympathetic efferent fibres that contain noradrenaline. It has been known for some considerable time that section of the sympathetic innervation of a part of the body suffering intractable pain often has a beneficial effect. Part of the reason for this is probably that unmyelinated sensory afferents run alongside the sympathetic fibres and are cut at the same time. It is, however, possible to show a more selective association of the sympathetic system and pain, for it has been found in clinical studies that adrenergic neurone blocking agents such as guanethidine will relieve the pain (causalgia) that is seen in some patients with peripheral nerve lesions. This is a complex area, but one that may be of great importance, and it will be seen later that substances related chemically to noradrenaline may have a role in modulating pain perception within the brain too.

Neurotransmitters within the central nervous system

Neurotransmission within the central nervous system has two possible functions, namely excitation or inhibition. These functions may be exerted in a direct way (now often thought of as classical neurotransmission), whereby synaptic release of a chemical messenger leads to activation or depression of neuronal activity in the manner of an on/off switch, or alternatively in a more subtle manner, which has been called modulation and which leads to an enabling or disenabling of neuronal responses to a pre-existing threshold input. Detailed discussion of these matters is outside the scope of this text, but all variations in the neurotransmission process are likely to be relevant to the subject of pain perception.

The first, and possibly the most crucial, site of chemical neurotransmission in the pain perception process is within the dorsal horn of the spinal cord. In particular, the possibility that functionally distinct nerve fibres may use different neurotransmitters raises the question of a selective pharmacological manipulation of sensory inputs.

It has been known for some time that glutamic acid and

structurally related acidic amino acids powerfully excite central neurones when applied in the vicinity of the single cell using appropriate microelectrode techniques. The dorsal horn is no exception to this rule, and an excitatory amino acid, possibly glutamic acid, is likely to be a transmitter released by larger, myelinated primary afferent fibres. The weight of evidence now suggests that most (if not all) fibres, large or small, use excitatory amino acid transmitters. Many small sensory afferents also contain peptides, and these may be the key to some of their special properties, including pain perception. In particular, the 11 amino acid peptide, substance P, mentioned earlier in the light of its possible peripheral functions, has received much study, and there is now good evidence that it is contained in and released by unmyelinated primary afferents. Patients suffering chronic pain have now been observed to have elevated levels of substance P in lumbar cerebrospinal fluid, although the precise significance of these data is not yet apparent, and some animal experiments consistently point to a specific role for substance P in nociception rather than other sensory modalities. Other peptides (for example vasoactive intestinal polypeptide and somatostatin) are also known to be present in small, unmyelinated afferent fibres, and in some cases may even coexist within the same fibre. This produces a most confusing picture, for it is not unreasonable to suppose that activity in a fibre with coexisting peptides would lead to the release of both peptides. However, there is some evidence from studies on autonomic efferents that two substances contained in the same nerve fibre can be released in either an independent fashion or together dependent on the frequency of impulse traffic in the fibre. The simplistic idea that substance P or some other small peptide is the 'pain transmitter' is not tenable in the light of our current knowledge, and it is likely that the coding of 'pain' within the dorsal horn involves a combination of neuromessenger substances.

At the present time less is known about the neurotransmitters involved in the transmission of messages from the dorsal horn to higher centres, but it is probable that both peptides and amino acids are involved.

Inhibitory neurotransmission is also important in determining whether or not tissue damage results in the experience of pain by an individual. Areas of the brainstem seem to be important in generating inhibition of nociceptive input and of the motor responses to such input via pathways descending to the dorsal and ventral horns of the spinal cord. Inhibition of sensory input also occurs locally within the dorsal horn of the spinal cord and at other relay nuclei on the way to the cerebral cortex. Although those inhibitory circuits can be demonstrated to exist by electrical stimulation of the relevant pathways, they can also be shown to be turned on by the type of tissue-damaging stimuli that give rise to pain and by other forms of stress. The neurotransmitter substances involved are many and varied. In the same way that it is true to say that there is no such thing as a 'pain transmitter' there is also no one substance that acts as an 'analgesia transmitter' either. Initial studies suggested that the monoamines 5-hydroxytryptamine and noradrenaline had an important role in controlling pain threshold, and more recently peptides have also been shown to be involved. In particular, a group of peptides, the endogenous opioids, have actions very similar to those of analgesic drugs related to morphine (*see later*). The study of processes involving these opioids has been much assisted by the availability of a specific antagonist, naloxone, which could be used to block the effects of synaptically released opioid peptide. Opoid-operated inhibitions have been demonstrated on sensory relay neurones in the brainstem and on motoneurones within the ventral horn.

Much remains to be discovered about neutrotransmitters and pain. This is a very important area from which most of our present information about how pain-killing drugs work has been derived, and it is certainly the field of endeavour from which many new drugs for the treatment of pain will come.

CHAPTER 3
Factors Affecting the Severity of Pain

Introduction

The amount of pain perceived by the postoperative patient is determined by the severity of the stimulus and the augmentation or suppression of the resultant nervous impulses by the higher centres or 'mind'. The severity of the stimulus is determined by the site of surgery, by the amount of tissue damage and subsequent inflammation, by the degree of tension or movement of the surrounding muscles or strength of contraction of smooth muscle, and by the degree of distension of tissues or hollow organs. Other complicating factors also contribute to postoperative pain, for example: damage to, or swelling of, nerves; ischaemia of a part due to external pressure from bandages or plaster of Paris or to arterial inadequacy from thrombus, embolus, or tissue oedema; nerve damage from overmeticulous dissection; or urinary retention.

The inevitable pain of surgery is increased by factors such as muscle tension and movement, anxiety or fear, fatigue and frustration, depression and disappointment, by other discomforts, and by the duration of the pain. Patients also differ from one another in respect of their pain threshold, i.e. the intensity of stimulation which is interpreted as pain, and in respect of their pain tolerance, i.e. the amount by which the stimulation must be increased before it is interpreted as intolerable or agonizing. The factors which affect pain threshold, pain tolerance, or the amount of analgesic required are anxiety, age, sex, race, and culture.

Site of operation

There is general agreement in analgesic studies that operations on the thorax and abdomen are more painful than operations on the skin, limbs, or even head. There are exceptions to this rule: for example, a phantom limb pain can be convulsively intolerable or an ischaemic limb following imperfect arterial surgery may be agonizing. Yet pain following operations on the limbs or body shell can be reduced by immobilizing the injured part, and sometimes the post-traumatic oedema can be reduced by elevating the damaged area. If the nerves within the injured tissue are stimulated less often or less severely, the threshold of those nerves, although lowered, will not be reached so frequently and the perceived pain will be less. Certainly the pain caused by the released algogenic substances described in Chapter 2, the lowered pain threshold of the receptors, and the pressure from the inflammatory swelling exacerbated by the increased blood flow, cannot be avoided, but severe pain caused by movement of the injured part can be avoided by splinting and by protection of its surface from further impact.

The chest or abdomen cannot be immobilized without reducing ventilation. The greatest ventilatory movement occurs, in most cases, in the ribs which form the lower costal margin, i.e. the 7th to the 10th. Upper abdominal and lower thoracic operations are therefore more painful than those in the lower abdomen or upper chest.

The size and direction of the incision also affects the severity of the pain, since this determines, in part, the amount of damaged tissue, the muscle spasm, and distribution of neural involvement. A unilateral vertical incision is usually less painful than a midline one, and a subcostal or intercostal incision less painful than a vertical one. It is likely that the degree of guarding of pleural, peritoneal, and intraperitoneal structures will be similar, but the pain caused by spasm of damaged muscles will be less when the involvement is unilateral, and less still when only one group of segmental muscles is pulling on the incision.

Pain arises not only from somatic structures such as skin, muscle, and the parietal pleura and peritoneum, but also from visceral structures such as the gastrointestinal tract, biliary and pancreatic tracts, ureters, etc. Visceral surgery often leads to uncoordinated smooth muscle contraction, which may be excessive and painful or lead to distension of the hollow viscus, which is also painful. This pain may be spasmodic or colicky, or may lead to hypersensitivity of the somatic structures within the same afferent nerve receptor field.

Pain not at the site of operation

Although postoperative pain is predominantly that of the operated site, there may be other conditions which exacerbate the operative pain or even exceed it. These may exist prior to the operative period, occur coincidentally during this time, or be a consequence of the operative management.

The pain may be referred from structures close to the operation to a distant site. Shoulder tip pain may occur as a result of irritation of structures around the diaphragm because of gas (e.g. laparoscopy) or inflammation (subphrenic abscess). Discomfort may arise from procedures which are part of the operative management, e.g. nasogastric drainage, catheter spasm, intravenous puncture, or infusion, especially when associated with haematoma or extravasation. It may arise as an expected or unexpected result of the anaesthetic management, e.g. sore throat, post-spinal headache, pneumothorax (say after central venous line placement). It may also be associated with postoperative state, the pain or the immobility, or even the narcotic medication to combat the pain. It can be caused by a full bladder, pressure sores, deep vein thrombosis, and pulmonary emboli.

Pain may also be due to conditions which existed prior to surgery and are unrelated to the presenting conditions. These can be made worse in the perioperative period. Some chronic pain conditions are relatively unchanged by surgery — trigeminal neuralgia, post-herpetic neuralgia, multiple sclerosis — and the pain may be eased by postoperative medication. Some conditions may be made worse by the operative management, e.g. chronic cervical or lumbar pain by bed rest, and arthritis if the usual oral anti-inflammatory analgesics are withheld. Renal calculi may be encouraged by the preoperative starvation and dehydration.

More serious are the conditions which are made worse by surgery or the stress of surgery. Angina pectoris or myocardial ischaemia may be made worse in stress or postoperative pain, recovery, or infection. The cardiac output rises, the heart rate rises, and the peripheral resistance rises. More work must be done by the myocardium against a greater resistance and with less time in diastole for relaxation and coronary artery perfusion. Myocardial infarction is thus most likely in conditions of stress, infection, and pain, especially during the recovery of consciousness. Migraine headaches may be precipitated by stress, not usually at the time of stress but following it. Sympathetic dystrophy or causalgia is also made worse by surgery unless sympathetic ablation is performed at the same time. The cause for this, as for sympathetic dystrophy, is unknown, but the original condition arises as a response to partial nerve damage or severe stress, and the pain occurs in the absence of stimulation and is made worse by local and circulating catecholamines, e.g. adrenaline. There is a rise in the level of catecholamines before and after surgery. All these conditions give rise to pain which may be eased by opiates but which may not be appropriately treated in this way.

How this pain is interpreted, and the reaction to this pain and to analgesics, depends very much on the personality of the patient and the situation in which the pain occurs. Factors such as age, sex, and sociocultural backgrounds influence greatly the perception, reaction, and expression of pain, but they are unlikely to be subject to modification within the hospital admission. Situational factors, such as anxiety about hospitals, operations, or pain, fatigue, loss of choice or independence, and loss of privacy or dignity, can often be modified by reassurance and evidence of caring and competence to minimize the experience of pain. This modification may be at least as important as analgesic drugs.

Age

The effect of age on the pain experience is not simple. On one hand, Procacci *et al.* (1974) reported a progressive increase of the pain threshold with age, on the other Woodrow *et al.* (1972) showed that older persons are more sensitive to pain. Certainly, the thickening of the skin with age increases the pain threshold of experimentally induced pricking or radiant heat pain, and certainly the effect of narcotic analgesics is increased with age, as is the sedation and lack of arousal by pain. The expression of pain, either in reactions or by facial expression, is less with age, but the threshold of pain and severe pain from a perceived stimulus has not been shown to be altered by age. However, the practical effect of age is considerable, in that the volume of distribution of the drug is lower, the clearance of analgesic drugs is slower, and optimal dose or frequency of dose is less. The aged patient is less tolerant of the side-effects of the drugs, such as narcosis, constipation, and, in the case of the local anaesthetics, depression of myocardial contraction. Neonates present problems which are discussed in Chapter 12.

Sex

The effect of sex on pain experience and expression is also subject to dispute. Studies of experimental radiant heat showed that the cutaneous pricking pain threshold is lower is women than in men. Furthermore, the threshold varies with the menstrual cycle, being greater in the first half of the cycle and less in the second. There is even a different response to narcotic analgesics. Postoperatively, Nayman (1979) found that females registered a higher average index of pain than males, but that the difference did not achieve significance ($p = 0.06$). In his study, the morphine infusion was adjusted by the nursing staff, and the males were given, on average, larger amounts of morphine. This, combined with the shorter elimination phase of morphine in females (*see below*), may account for the difference.

Body weight

Obesity is considered in Chapter 12.

Race and cultural background

In general, Mediterranean peoples are more demonstrative, expressive, and demanding when in pain than the northern European. In turn, the Scandinavian demands less pain relief than the Anglo-Saxon. It has also been reported that Orientals and Negroes are more sensitive than average Caucasians to experimental pain (Woodrow *et al.* 1972), but conversely that Chinese, Filipinos and Japanese need fewer analgesics than Caucasians (Streltze & Wade 1981). It is probable that the way of life is also important in determining the pain threshold and tolerance. It was found that Nepalese Sherpas had an abnormally low sensitivity to pain, yet the families and relatives of those Sherpas living in lowland villages had pain sensitivities within the normal range.

Personality and social conditioning

Anxiety increases the severity of the pain experience and is considered below. Depression too, possibly by concentrating the thoughts on the pain, misery, and implications of the pain, increases the pain suffered although, because of reduced spontaneous expression, this suffering may not be obvious. Conversely, those with pain associated with a life-threatening or mutilating condition, or those with pain of long duration, are likely to be depressed.

Extroversion and emotionality alter the pain experience. Some people say that they feel things more deeply, more 'acutely', or more severely, than most. If they are uninhibited in their reaction to pain, stress or other experiences, this may well be true. Strong emotion such as excitement, horror, or intense pleasure inhibits pain. Extroverts are less inhibited in expressing their pain. The swings from discomfort towards agony tend to be wider, and they are more likely to complain of pain (Parbrook et al. 1973). Thus their pain scores tend to be higher and they receive more analgesics. In general, neurotics have the same pain threshold as normal, but the reaction is abnormal. The pain threshold of lobotomized subjects is also unchanged, but the reaction is little or none.

In the same way as the extrovert is rewarded for his expression of pain by increased analgesic administration, pain reaction or behaviour varies with the situation, company, and expectation of response. The complaint of pain may be made when the desired aim is company, sympathy, reassurance, or sleep. Pain is an expected event following surgery, and one which the patient and staff expect to be treated. Fear and loneliness may be felt as deeply but engender less sympathy and attention from the attendants.

The complaint of pain may vary with the company. It is a common experience that a patient who has just refused analgesia complains to an attentive spouse/relative/friend that he has been in unrelieved pain.

A patient in pain may deny or choose not to complain of his pain. This may be because of the side-effects of the analgesia, e.g. confusion, nausea, or loss of function, or because of shame or because the expectation of pain relief is low. Pain is still, consciously or unconsciously, regarded by some as a judgement or penalty for sins committed and to be borne without complaint. This is especially so in pain involving the sexual organs or perineum. In others, it is an embarrassment to mention or complain of pain in such parts. The complaint of pain may represent the loss of pride or virility, and this attitude is still, unfortunately, voiced occasionally by the medical or nursing staff. Other patients may not wish to trouble the nursing/medical staff, preferring to suffer pain rather than be thought a nuisance, and this is exaggerated when the attendants appear to be busy or are unattentive, or when the complaint is superficially trivial or the cause of possible merriment, e.g. cramp, haemorrhoids.

Patients may have a poor expectation of pain relief. A postoperative questionnaire (Campbell 1977) revealed that 48% of patients were unaware that pain relief was readily available, and most patients had to request pain relief themselves. In many cases analgesic drugs are delayed for the convenience of the routine of the ward, and in many others there is a considerable delay before two unoccupied nurses of sufficient rank can be found to administer analgesic drugs. If the nursing staff are obviously busy or occupied in conversation or medical reports on or off the ward, a request for analgesia may not be made.

Anxiety before and after operation

The stress reaction is a pattern of physiological and psychological changes in an individual under threat of danger or unwanted circumstances. Anxiety is one of these changes. Persistent anxiety and stress may have their own debilitating effects.

Simple admission to hospital, with its known and unknown implications, causes anxiety and physiological changes such as tachycardia, hypertension, sweating, and increased muscle tone. This state varies considerably from one individual to another. Many studies have shown that the severity of anxiety preoperatively correlates well with the amount of postoperative pain and the incidence of pulmonary complications following abdominal surgery. Others (e.g. Chapman 1985) have shown that pain levels correlate well with anxiety over the days of *recovery* from elective abdominal surgery.

Anxiety is caused or increased by a number of factors. Norris and Baird (1967) examined 300 patients preoperatively and classified 60% as anxious. More women than men showed anxiety. Fear was predominantly about general health (31%), operation (38%), and uncertainty of the results (26%). Some expressed fear of the anaesthetic (17%) and of postoperative pain (12%). Others feared the loss of dignity, such as possible catheterization for urinary retention, bowel problems, and even preoperative shaving. A very common fear is that related to the lack of knowledge of the surgical and nursing procedures. When mutilation or death is a possible outcome of surgery, anxiety is greater. This is seen especially before diagnostic laparotomy for possible malignancy, mastectomy, and where colostomy or amputation is the possible result of surgery.

A feeling of helplessness also increases stress and muscle tension. The patient no longer has control over the operation or the results. He is not allowed to make many decisions which form part of his normal life, including that of analgesic intake, independent movement, choice of food, and so on. Patients may be seen to demonstrate disappointment on hearing phrases such as 'not now', 'I'm busy', 'it's not our policy' or 'you have had all you are allowed', phrases which diminish the patient as an individual and make him less important than a rule or routine. A seemingly uncaring attitude towards one patient induces stress in others who are made aware, by example, of their own vulnerability. Unfortunately, some patients tend to exaggerate the severity of their operation or disability or discomfort when relating their experiences, and this too will induce anxiety in other patients.

Most patients admit to some anxiety prior to surgery, and by their admission cope with the fear and distress of the operation and postoperative result and discomfort. Others have excessive fear or panic, and the changes in heart rate and blood pressure may represent a risk to health. Yet others cope with fear by denying that it exists and show no anxiety at all. Explanation of the operation and personal experience interferes with the denier's ability to cope and *increases* stress. The law, however, demands that *informed* consent is obtained before operation; this includes information of common side-effects or complications. A denier is also less able to cope with the stress of any complication or unexpected outcome and, on balance, the optimum approach is to combine information with reassurance where possible.

Chapter 3

Psychological preparation for surgery

The stress of hospital admission can be reduced by giving adequate notice of that admission, so that domestic affairs, e.g. child-minding, sick leave, etc., can be ordered. With that notice of admission should be sent a leaflet giving information on the hospital and that which is expected of the patient. This will include a map of the hospital and how to get there, bus stops and car parking if any, the entrance through which one should enter, how to get to the admission desk, directions to the ward for the patient and visitors, what clothing and money to bring, the expected duration of stay including that before operation, the hours of visiting, and the hours in which it is convenient for telephone enquiries.

Some hospitals in some specialties, for example obstetrics and paediatric surgery, allow the patients to visit the hospital and the departments in which they will be treated before the date of admission or confinement. In paediatric surgery, studies have been made of the effect of showing a film of the proposed conscious experience compared to the effect of showing an unrelated film. Those children who saw a realistic film of what they were about to undergo showed fewer anxiety-related behaviour patterns and less disturbance on the night before surgery than the others. They also showed less sleep disturbance, fewer tantrums, and less bed-wetting in the weeks after surgery. The film must be realistic, and the subject of the film must demonstrate anxiety which is reduced by reassurance and by demonstration and explanation throughout the procedure. If the film subject can cope with his anxiety, the patient watching the film can cope better also. If the film subject shows no anxiety or no discomfort on venepuncture, the patient cannot identify with the subject and the advantage is lost. Similar demonstrations, sometimes called 'peer-modelling', can be adopted with colostomy, mastectomy, or amputation, whereby the patient can be reassured by another who has experienced the procedure and has coped with the problems.

On admission, the patient must be made to feel welcome and allowed to retain as much personal identity and dignity as possible. The hospital admitting clerk should not be remote and protected from the patient. For example, if a counter is used, it should be open rather than protected by glass partitions so that eye and hand contact is possible; it should resemble that of a hotel foyer rather than that a bank. A smile and a handshake is important to a patient who is fearful of being depersonalized to a number or a case history. Similarly, patients should be greeted on the ward by the ward staff, and shown rather than directed to a bed. The bed should be identified by the patient's name in large letters so that thereafter the patient can be addressed by name rather than such epithets as 'love', 'ducks' or 'dear', which, although meant well or with affection, are regarded by some as demeaning. Courtesy demonstrated to a patient suggests a caring and efficient attitude of the staff and engenders confidence in the patient: it costs little in time or effort and is rewarded by the increased ability of the patient to cope with pain or disability, by fewer complications, and possibly a shortened hospital stay. Discourtesy or aggression on the part of the patient is likely to be a symptom of anxiety and requires a more, not less, caring attitude.

Adequate explanation of the operation, procedures, and tests should be given by the medical staff and should include the personal conscious experience of the patient. This should always be accompanied by the reassurance that care will be taken to minimize the occurrence of side-effects or complications, which will be treated if necessary. The patient should be told, for example, that some postoperative pain is to be expected following abdominal surgery (if local anaesthetic techniques are not used), but that it will be minimized so that breathing and limb movements are comfortable, and that additional analgesia is available if necessary by regular administration, by request, or by self-administration. He should be shown how to cough, and how to move so as to avoid the pain of sudden movement. It is known that general explanation without reassurance is not effective in reducing anxiety and muscle tone, whereas a full explanation combined with reassurance reduces both and minimizes the amount of analgesics required postoperatively. It is well established that the preoperative visit by the anaesthetist is at least as effective in alleviating anxiety as premedicant drugs. It is important to describe the place of recovery of consciousness and to explain the equipment that may be attached to the patient, e.g. nasogastric tubes, intravenous infusion, drains, etc. Those patients who wake up in the recovery room or intensive therapy unit with unexpected monitoring or treatment lines attached are likely to assume that the operation has gone disastrously wrong. Similarly, it is helpful to reassure the patient who is coming out of unconsciousness, perhaps into pain, that the operation has, in fact, finished. It is now the practice in some hospitals for theatre or anaesthetic room nurses to visit the patient preoperatively. This is especially reassuring, since the patient will feel that there are staff who are caring during the period of unconsciousness. The patient should never feel abandoned, and it is preferable that a ward nurse accompanies him to theatre and remains until he is asleep. The physiotherapist can be especially helpful before operation, not only by training the patient to breathe effectively and showing how the discomfort, if any, of coughing can be minimized, but also by teaching muscle relaxation. This is also effective in reducing postoperative pain and muscle tension.

A patient may be fearful that he may waken during the operation, feeling pain but paralysed and unable to communicate. The mention of this unlikely event by the medical or nursing staff may cause unwarranted anxiety. If it is voiced by the patient, perhaps in response to some film or television thriller or to articles in the medical press, he should be offered the isolated arm technique. By this method, a tourniquet is applied to one arm and inflated prior to and for several minutes after the injection of the muscle relaxant. He or she can then be reassured that should consciousness occur, communicating signals may be made with that arm.

Avoidance of fatigue

Although there is no unequivocal evidence that shows pain to be increased by fatigue, it is a common experience that fatigue reduces tolerance and the ability to concentrate (and thereby be distracted from pain) and increases confusion. Sleep increases the sensory threshold to pain. Fatigue can be due to the loss of sleep preoperatively because of anxiety or to the loss of sleep before and after operation because of strange or excessive noise (tea trolleys, excited conversation, admission of new patients or theatre trolleys for emergency operations). Loss of sleep may occur after surgery because of enthusiastic monitoring of the blood pressure, urinary drainage, etc. Monitoring of the pulse rate and volume can be performed without waking a patient and will indicate changes in blood flow and pressure. An automatic blood pressure recording device or intra-arterial monitors cause less disturbance than the manual method. Monitoring of the respiratory rate and depth gives an early indication not only of respiratory distress or chest complications but also, after thoracic or abdominal surgery, indicates the presence of pain or narcotic respiratory depression. It should be remembered that during sleep the respiratory rate is low, and rates of 12–14 per minute are not abnormal. If a patient is disturbed from sleep by these observations, the pulse, respiratory rate, and blood pressure may rise to abnormal levels and give false warnings of disease.

It is not unreasonable to make available a short-acting hypnotic, e.g. temazepam, the night before surgery should the patient be unable to sleep because of anxiety or strange noises or because he is disturbed by the ward activities.

Problems of existing narcotic dependence and abuse

The problems of the patient who habitually takes large doses of narcotic analgesics (usually an opioid) in a controlled way, say for painful terminal disease, are those of drug tolerance and physical dependence. Psychic dependence is unusual. Adequate narcotic analgesia must be given continuously or at regular intervals to prevent withdrawal and to treat the existing pain. Narcotic analgesics may also be required for the superimposed postoperative pain, and often in increased amounts. Very large amounts may be required. Six grams per day of diamorphine or morphine are occasionally taken by terminally ill patients without any detectable signs of ventilatory depression. Most partial agonists can precipitate the withdrawal syndrome and should not be used. If it is not possible to provide continuous or regular analgesia, long-acting analgesics, such as methadone, can be substituted. Postoperatively, the rate of absorption from the usual site of administration may be reduced (gastric stasis, regional hypoperfusion), and the analgesic rendered temporarily or relatively ineffective. The dose, frequency, and site can be altered, and the intravenous route is the most reliable.

The chronic drug abuser presents additional problems. The drug intake is probably variable, depending on the ethics of the drug pusher, and there is usually considerable psychic dependence and fear of withdrawal. The patient is likely to be very demanding of analgesics, even to the point of injury to himself or to the staff. The purity of illegal drugs is variable, and either drug overdose or drug withdrawal may present on admission to hospital. Because of the drug tolerance and physical dependence, the high drug levels must be maintained to prevent withdrawal symptoms during the postoperative period. The variable standards of sterility, and contamination of the drugs, injection equipment, and site of injection, combined with personal neglect of hygiene and food intake, increase the probabilities of systemic disease, hepatic damage, and difficulty of venous access.

Postoperative analgesia is best achieved by regional anaesthesia whenever possible. Continuous infusion of opioids is a logical approach to postoperative pain relief and to the maintenance of habitual opioid levels. Any such device should be tamperproof, and small reservoirs of drug should be used. Patient-controlled analgesia is a technique which is not very suitable for these patients.

As the postoperative pain declines, efforts should be made to withdraw the narcotic analgesic. Most authorities favour the substitution of methadone. An equally valid approach is to reduce the strength of the injections while maintaining their volume and frequency. If medication is by mouth, the drug should be dissolved in flavoured, coloured syrup, and the strength of the drug reduced while maintaining the strength of the flavour and colour and volume of the linctus.

The reformed addict is also a problem in that pain tolerance remains low for years after drug addiction and the patient is more likely to become addicted on challenge with narcotic analgesics. As before, regional anaesthesia should be used if possible, but, if not possible, systemic analgesics should be used in full and appropriate strength to relieve the pain, and drug withdrawal started as soon as possible after the postoperative pain has resolved.

Many of the features of opioid withdrawal (painful spasms in the abdomen and calves, vomiting, diarrhoea, pyrexia, hypertension or hypotension) mimic those of complications of surgery. Agitation is usually more pronounced than is usual for a similar surgical complication, and the patient often asks for medication by name. The abstinence syndrome is often eased by drugs such as clonidine or chlorpromazine. Postoperative hypotension may be a sign of bleeding, or of drug overdose or withdrawal, or of adrenal suppression combined with postoperative stress. Adrenocorticosteroids may be needed. Pregnant patients are more likely to go into premature labour when the level of requirement of their narcotic analgesic changes. Pethidine is a stimulant of uterine muscle in late pregnancy and morphine a suppressant. The infant will have not only the problems of immaturity, but those of narcotic withdrawal.

Summary

Many factors influence the incidence and severity of postoperative pain. Some factors, like the site of operation, the feasibility of immobilizing the injured part, and predisposing factors, such as age, sex, and racial and cultural learned behaviour, cannot be altered within a hospital admission. Other factors, such as excessive retractor pressure or tissue damage, prolonged ischaemia, and especially anxiety, also increase the postoperative analgesic requirement, and these can be minimized.

CHAPTER 4

Consequences of Postoperative Pain

The humanitarian desire to relieve postoperative pain is sometimes overridden by the fear of depression of the respiratory, cardiovascular, or central nervous systems by narcotic analgesics, or of hypotension, pneumothorax, etc. caused by local anaesthetic techniques, or of other side-effects of the analgesic drugs. The diversion of staff time, effort, and expertise, and of equipment and drugs, to the provision of optimal analgesia is not generally feasible. However, optimal analgesia not only improves the quality of life in the postoperative period, it reduces the incidence of complications, the degree of pre- and postoperative stress, and the time required to be spent in hospital. The expenditure of time and equipment for analgesia is probably cost-effective.

The retrospective analysis of a feasibility study of epidural opioid analgesia for biliary surgery showed that 20 patients in the epidural group had a postoperative hospital stay of two days less than the 18 similar patients who had intermittent narcotic injections on demand. The change in attitude of nursing, anaesthetic, and surgical staff has made it impossible to reproduce the previous conditions within the control group.

Complications of postoperative pain are due to the body's reaction to pain or to its efforts to avoid further pain. This pain does not have to be appreciated at a conscious level: the fixed facial expression, the truncated respiratory pattern, the immobility of the body persist into sleep. It is well known that powerful stimuli such as anal dilation can cause bronchoconstriction, laryngospasm, and changes in blood pressure and muscle movement in patients who are in the surgical planes of anaesthesia and who would not react to incision and other surgical manipulation. Pain responses do not always depend upon the conscious appreciation of a noxious stimulus. They can, however, be eliminated by analgesics or local anaesthetics.

Pain leads not only to guarding of muscles around the area of pain, but to muscle rigidity distant from that site. The flatness of facial expression, or even grimacing, and immobility of trunk and limbs are examples. Vasoconstriction and pallor occur throughout the body. Immobility and venous stasis lead to venous thrombosis, pressure sores, and urinary calculi. Venous thrombosis may lead to pulmonary emboli. Massive pulmonary embolus is the commonest cause of sudden death in the first 10 days after surgery. Kakkar *et al.* (1975), showed that pulmonary embolus was responsible for 16% of all postoperative deaths in general surgical patients over the age of 40 in whom no special prophylactic measures had been taken. Other predisposing factors include obesity, long duration of surgical procedure, upper abdominal operations and prostatectomy, pancreatitis, and the contraceptive pill.

Pulmonary complications

The clinical syndrome known as 'the postoperative chest', which includes pyrexia, tachycardia, dyspnoea, chest pain, purulent sputum, and auscultatory and radiological changes, is most common after upper abdominal surgery, much less common after lower abdominal surgery, and rare after surgery on the limbs and body surface. It is less common after mid-thoracic than upper abdominal surgery. The factors which predispose towards this syndrome are acute and chronic bronchitis (especially from smoking), obesity, and pain. Those with chronic bronchitis and bronchorrhoea can be improved by withdrawal of tobacco and intensive physiotherapy preoperatively so that the overall perioperative change is small. The obese patient is at risk in many respects — difficult surgical, venous, and airway access, regurgitation and aspiration, venous thrombosis, and pulmonary mechanical and vascular difficulties — and should be encouraged to lose weight if at all possible. However, the low incidence of the postoperative chest following limb and body surface surgery suggests that the principal problem is abdominal pain, muscle spasm, and other factors which restrict the diaphragm and lung movement. Similarly, although transvesical prostatectomy carries a moderately high risk of pulmonary complications, transurethral procedures do not.

Mechanism of postoperative pulmonary complications and hypoxaemia

There are many valid reasons for hypoxaemia immediately after operation: diffusion hypoxia of nitrous oxide, increased ventilation–perfusion imbalance, accumulation of secretion, reflex bronchoconstriction, and accidental aspiration during anaesthesia. These would be independent of site of operation. Hypoxaemia after 24 hours is relatively independent of the anaesthetic used and varies with the site of operation, being worse after upper abdominal surgery. The pain of the abdominal incision and peritoneal inflammation is accompanied by spasm or guarding of the muscles of the abdominal wall. These muscles, the rectus transversus abdominis and internal and external oblique, are muscles of forced expiration. Their contraction increases the abdominal pressure, raises the diaphragm, increases the transpulmonary pressure, and forces gas out of the lungs. Their sustained contraction maintains a reduction in the size of the lungs throughout normal tidal ventilation. The pressure on the airways is greater, and the airways tend to collapse earlier in expiration or even remain closed throughout tidal ventilation (Alexander *et al.* 1973). This increases the ventilation–perfusion imbalance, causing shunting of pulmonary arterial blood through unventilated lung tissue. The greater the degree of airway closure throughout tidal volume, the longer the shunt. These changes reduce the uptake of oxygen by the blood. This postoperative hypoxaemia can be treated by increasing the inspired concentration of oxygen, but the greater the extent of the shunt, the less effect the increased inspired oxygen will have. This problem is worse in the bronchitic and the aged, where loss of lung elasticity has increased the closing capacity, and in the obese and those with pneumothorax or intraperitoneal gas, where the resting lung volume (FRC) is reduced. The gas distal to the site of prolonged airway closure is absorbed and pulmonary collapse results. This, in itself, can cause pain. The further reduction in lung size and area for gas exchange causes further hypoxaemia, confusion, or narcosis, and some patients progress to pneumonia and/or respiratory failure.

Other factors which predispose to this problem are the head-down position, frequently adopted for hypotension, abdominal binders, deep tension sutures, gastric dilatation, and acute distension of the bladder. Late pregnancy has been shown to increase airway closure in the sitting position. Pneumothoraces should be drained routinely, and gas within the abdomen, introduced inevitably during laparotomy or deliberately during laparoscopy, can also be drained; this reduces the incidence of pain following laparoscopy (Alexander & Hull 1987). Copious and viscous sputum is retained if the ability to cough is reduced because of thoracic or abdominal pain. Yet the presence of respiratory distress is frequently taken as an indication to withold narcotic analgesics, as is the presence of chronic obstructive airway disease. Increasing hypoxaemia or hypercarbia because of adequate narcotic analgesics is an indication for local anaesthetic techniques. If they too cause respiratory failure or are inappropriate, and if other techniques such as opioid—ketamine analgesia are ineffective, postoperative analgesia should be provided during intermittent positive-pressure ventilation.

Effects of pain on ventilation

If breathing is painful, deep breathing is more so. The ventilation becomes shallow, and the carbon dioxide tension, the respiratory drive, and the ventilatory rate increase. While rapid shallow ventilation is capable of eliminating carbon dioxide, it is relatively inefficient for taking up oxygen. The hypoxaemia, from this and other reasons, increases the respiratory drive and ventilatory rate, and reduces the carbon dioxide further. The respiratory alkalosis opposes the shift of the oxygen dissociation curve produced by hypoxic tissues and tends to retain oxygen in the blood rather than in the tissues. The respiratory alkalosis is compensated for by the renal elimination of bicarbonate. More carbon dioxide dissolves, lowering the carbon dioxide further. Conversely, the ventilatory drive is maintained by the pain via the reticular activating system. If the pain is relieved, and if narcotic analgesics are administered, or even if sleep supervenes, the respiratory drive may be inadequate, and apnoea or Cheyne—Stokes ventilation may occur. It follows that oscillations between pain and analgesia are more dangerous than continuous analgesia.

The hypocarbia also causes vasoconstriction, which further decreases the flow of oxygen to the tissues. This may reduce wound healing and causes cerebral hypoxia and confusion.

The metabolic consequences of postoperative pain

There are many changes in hormonal levels or metabolism in response to anaesthesia and surgery (Moore & McQuay 1985). Not all of these are wholly or partly in response to pain. Some are increased by opioid agonists or anaesthetic gases, which reduce the amount of perceived pain. Others decline or do not persist in the postoperative period even when pain is present. The significance of these changes is uncertain, and the more basic question — are these changes beneficial or detrimental to the patient? — is still unanswered.

The changes in carbohydrate, nitrogen, and fat balance promote a high plasma glucose level and an available source of energy for the glucose-dependent organs such as the brain and heart. They also cause decreased peripheral utilization of glucose and mobilization of glucose from amino acids and peripheral fat. This leads to an excessive breakdown of protein tissue, osteoporosis, and a negative nitrogen balance. The decreased glucose tolerance promotes an osmotic diuresis. The changes in water balance are those which increase reabsorption of sodium and increase or maintain the extracellular volume at the expense of excretion of potassium and hydrogen ions. The alkalosis so caused opposes the acidosis produced during the postoperative starvation by the mobilization of fat. These changes have an evolutionary advantage to any wounded animal which would be deprived of food and water. They may have less benefit for those patients in a standard postoperative ward where calories and fluid are available.

The level of glucose and of nitrogen breakdown is governed by the hormones of the pituitary and gonads, and by adrenaline and hormones of the adrenal cortex. The fluid balance and size of the extracellular volume is controlled by the antidiuretic hormone and aldosterone.

Anterior pituitary hormones

Although prolactin and growth hormone are increased in concentration many-fold during anaesthesia and surgery, the increase declines after the end of the operation despite persistence of pain. Although the rise in prolactin levels is reduced by extensive spinal anaesthesia, it is increased by opioids. The rise in concentration of growth hormone is reduced not only by spinal anaesthesia, but also by large doses of fentanyl, and also by naloxone, an opioid antagonist (see p. 66).

Luteinizing hormone levels are raised in major but not minor surgery, and remain raised for several days. This increase is reduced by morphine analgesia but increased by ketamine analgesia. The correlation with pain therefore remains uncertain.

Adrenocorticotrophic hormone (ACTH)

There is a considerable rise in cortisol levels during surgery and the postoperative period, and this is presumed to be a result of raised ACTH levels. Also, it is known that stress, which includes pain, may induce analgesia through the release of beta-endorphin, which is released, molecule for molecule, with ACTH. However, although beta-endorphin can produce profound, prolonged analgesia when injected into the central nervous system, the plasma levels in stress are likely to have little effect and may reflect release from the active site or be a by-product of ACTH release. Promelanotropin is increased during surgery, and this enhances the adrenal responses to ACTH.

Sex hormones

Testosterone levels are reduced by anaesthesia, but are reduced even more during the postoperative period despite the raised levels of prolactin and luteinizing hormone. Since testosterone promotes nitrogen retention, perhaps by competition with the glucocorticoids, the lowered level may be a cause of the negative nitrogen balance.

Insulin, adrenaline, glucagon, and cortisol

Insulin

Plasma insulin concentrations do not change markedly after surgery except that of Caesarian section. However, the uptake of insulin by the cell is reduced, as is the plasma insulin response to a standard intravenous glucose infusion. The secretion of insulin is also inhibited by raised levels of adrenaline. These factors contribute to a persistent hyperglycaemia.

Glucagon

Glucagon levels are also raised postoperatively, the effect of which is to increase glucose production and increase peripheral glucose utilization. The level of glucagon can be increased by a persistently raised concentration of cortisol.

Adrenaline

The levels of adrenaline and, to a lesser extent, noradrenaline are raised significantly by preoperative anxiety and by laryngoscopy and intubation. They are raised also by postoperative anxiety and pain. Extradural anaesthesia from T4 to S5 inhibits the adrenaline response to surgery.

The rise in the level of secretion of adrenaline by the adrenal medulla is not necessarily linked to that of the endogenous adrenal opioid, alpha-neo-endorphin, plasma levels and analgesic effects of which are also raised postoperatively. Reserpine depletes the body of adrenaline and noradrenaline, but increases the plasma level of this opioid.

Cortisol

The cortisol concentration rises following the start of surgery, and this rise increases with the severity of the surgical stimulus, i.e. it changes little with body surface surgery or most neurosurgical procedures and considerably during thoracoabdominal operations. The increases are greater in women than in men. The plasma levels are raised during the first postoperative week following major surgery. Similar persistent increases are seen following trauma, the size of the increase again related to the severity of the trauma. Afferent nerve blockade by epidural local anaesthesia or epidural opioid analgesia can abolish the cortisol response to lower abdominal surgery, but that to upper abdominal surgery can be abolished only by spinal (subarachnoid or epidural) anaesthetic blockade involving the segments T4–S5.

Furthermore, although epidural opioid injections produce much more effective pain relief of the wound than intramuscular injections, the levels of cortisol (and adrenaline) are not significantly lower.

One must conclude that for pain relief to be effective in

abolishing the stress response to pain, it must be complete and involve the visceral afferents as well as those from the wound site.

Etomidate infusions preoperatively and as sedation in the intensive therapy unit reduce or abolish the cortisol response. Prolonged etomidate infusions result in increased mortality in severely ill patients. Buprenorphine given after total hip replacement produces a significant reduction in the postoperative cortisol increase in women but not in men. Meptazinol premedication is associated with a significantly higher plasma beta-endorphin level, and therefore ACTH levels, during operation under subarachnoid anaesthesia than is morphine premedication. The significance of these findings is unknown.

The interaction of these hormones can be summarized. Glucagon increases glucose synthesis and glucose utilization. Adrenaline increases glucose production transiently but decreases glucose utilization. Cortisol enhances the duration of the effects of adrenaline and glucagon, and a persistently high level of cortisol raises the concentration of glucagon. The resistance to the effect of insulin reduces the uptake of glucose by the cells. The hyperglycaemia leads to glycosuria, which is exaggerated by a lowered renal threshold.

This glucose synthesis is at the expense of body stores of fat and protein. Urinary nitrogen excretion is above normal for 4—5 days after major surgery, and this increased nitrogen loss can also be reduced by extensive prolonged extradural anaesthesia.

The effect of postoperative pain on fluid balance

Fluid balance is controlled by antidiuretic hormone and aldosterone, by the fluid intake, and by the osmolality of the glomerular filtrate. Renin may be increased during surgery, but restoration of renin release by epidural analgesia has no effect on postoperative diuresis or sodium excretion compared to general anaesthesia. Antidiuretic hormone (ADH) or 8-arginine vasopressin acts on the distal tubule of the nephron, the cortical and medullary collecting duct, to increase its permeability to water. In dehydration and in response to haemorrhage, pain, emotional stress, and pyrexia, the level of ADH rises and the urine decreases in volume and increases in osmolality. ADH responds quickly to such a stimulus, newly synthesized hormone being present in the posterior lobe of the pituitary within 30 minutes. Morphine causes oliguria, but it is thought that it inhibits ADH secretion by raising the osmotic threshold for release and that the oliguria is caused by an effect on the kidney or general circulation. The ADH rise in the operative and postoperative period can be blocked by extradural anaesthesia (T4–S5) and by high-dose epidural fentanyl. It is, however, possible that morphine has a separate ADH-releasing effect when applied to the brainstem.

In studies of ADH secretion after surgery where pain is controlled by epidural anesthesia, extradural morphine analgesia, and a combination of the two, the ADH levels were seen to rise after morphine injection, even in the group whose pain was already abolished. Furthermore, the delay in the rise of ADH levels after extradural morphine injection suggests that the effect of morphine was at the brainstem rather than on the spinal afferent impulses or via the circulation.

The adrenaline response to pain has a mixed effect on ADH secretion. The alpha-adrenergic effect is to cause a diuresis and the beta effect is to oppose it. Adrenergic drugs probably act primarily through the baroreceptor mechanism of ADH secretion.

The other effects of ADH, those on arterioles and other smooth muscle and on blood coagulation, are not usually significant at the levels found postoperatively. ADH is also associated with memory, with diurnal rhythms, and with morphine tolerance. It has corticotrophin releasing properties. The significance of these factors in the postoperative period and in postoperative disorientation is unknown.

Mineralocorticoids act on the distal tubule of the kidney to aid reabsorption of sodium ions and to increase the urinary excretion of potassium and hydrogen ions, leading to expansion of the extracellular fluid volume (ECF), hypokalaemia, and alkalosis. Lack of mineralocorticoids leads to sodium deficiency, shrinkage of the ECF and overhydration of cells, and to fits, circulatory collapse, renal failure, and death. Patients with chronic mineralocorticoid deficiency (Addison disease) exhibit apathy, depression, irritability, and sometimes psychosis. Aldosterone is raised during surgery and during the postoperative period. Anaesthesia alone has no effect on it. The aldosterone response can, however, be abolished by widespread extradural anaesthesia (T4–S5).

Conclusions

Although the stress response, including the response to pain, has evolved, presumably, with benefit to the organism, essential glucose-dependent functions are maintained at the expense of peripheral utilization of glucose and tissue breakdown and nitrogen loss. Thirst and the effect of the osmotic diuresis are opposed by sodium retention, but at the price of alkalosis, hypokalaemia, and oedema. In normal postoperative practice, the stress response can be reduced by reducing the stress that is perceived, i.e. by blocking the afferent stimulus by widespread spinal anaesthesia or potent spinal opioid analgesia. These procedures are associated with greater comfort, decreased morbidity, and earlier discharge from hospital. However, if the stress response is reduced but the perceived stress remains, as in Addison disease, steroid dependence, and, possibly, during etomidate infusions, then morbidity and mortality increase.

CHAPTER 5
The Pharmacology of Opioid Analgesics

Introduction

Opioids are the oldest and still the most useful class of drugs for the treatment of severe pain. Opium was known to the ancient civilizations of Egypt, Sumeria, and Babylon. It has been used for its ability to relieve pain, coughing, and diarrhoea, and to promote dreaming. It owes these actions to its content of morphine, and to a lesser extent other substances such as codeine. Morphine, codeine, and semisynthetic derivatives such as heroin are called opiates. The generic term opioid is used to describe the receptors

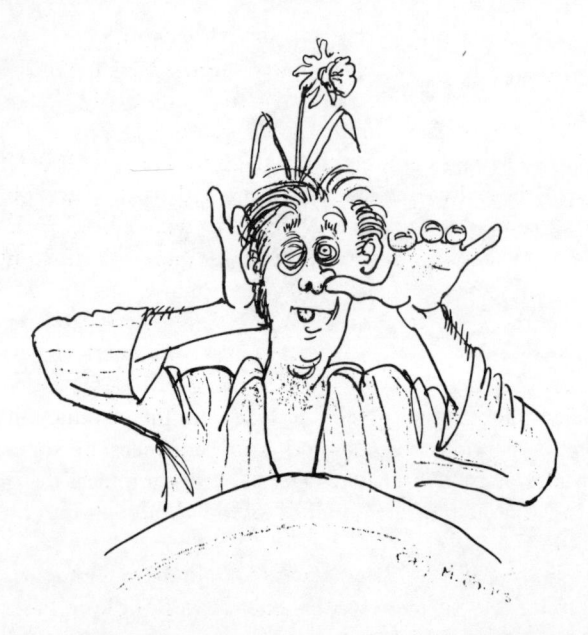

All opioids can lead to clouding of consciousness.

at which opiate drugs act, and also covers naturally occurring peptides and totally synthetic drugs such as pethidine and methadone. Thus, opioid drugs act at opioid receptors. All of the drugs named so far are agonists. There are also opioid antagonists, the best known being naloxone, which will prevent or reverse the action of the agonists. This substance is used to define the actions of a drug as truly opioid (largely due to the influence of Hans Kosterlitz), and only those actions which are reversed by naloxone should be so classified. This is particularly important for drugs with a wide range of actions, and morphine for instance can have non-opioid actions at receptors for inhibitory amino acids and acetylcholine. It is only recently that we have gained a clear understanding of how these agents work to relieve pain, and of why drugs in this general class have a wide range of actions that are unconnected to the relief of pain.

Endogenous opioid peptides

The discovery that analgesia produced by electrical stimulation of the rat brainstem could be reversed by naloxone, and the observation that radioactively labelled opioids would bind to discretely located sites in the brain, led to a search for naturally occurring opioids. The first success in this field was the isolation of the enkephalins by Hughes and his colleagues (*see* Hughes 1983). The discovery of these two pentapeptides has led to the subsequent isolation of some 18 endogenous peptides with opioid actions. Most (if not all) of these peptides belong to one of three families (*see* Fig. 5.1): the enkephalins, the endorphins, and the dynorphins. The precursors for each of these families are genetically distinct. Their amino acid sequences have been determined (by recombinant DNA analysis of their messenger RNAs), and proteolytic cleavage of the precursor leads to the production of active opioid peptides. The amino acid sequences of some of these peptides are shown in Table 5.1. The geographical distribution of the opioid peptide families in the brain of the rat is illustrated in Fig. 5.2.

In the brain the major endorphin-containing system starts in the arcuate nucleus of the hypothalamus, and from here projects to many areas of the brain, and possibly also to the spinal cord. A

Pro-opiomelanocortin

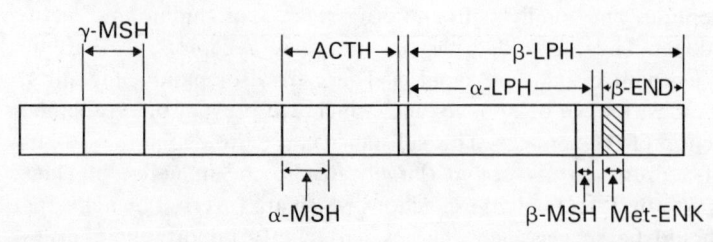

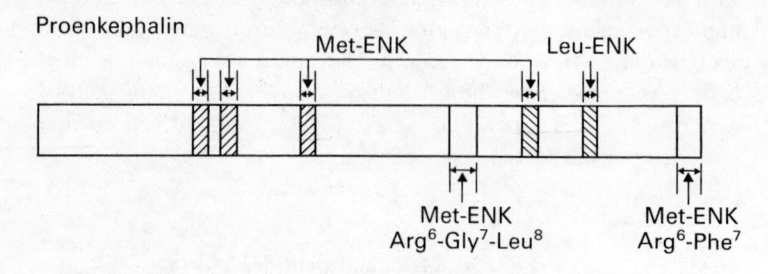

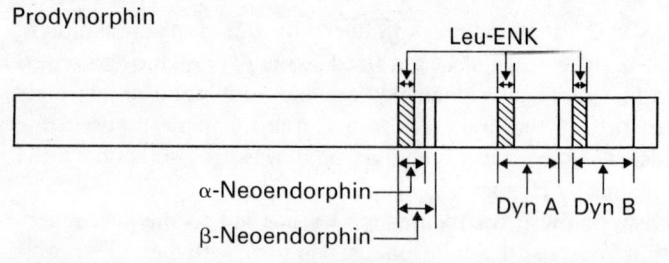

Fig. 5.1. Schematic representation of the structures of the protein precursors of the three families of opioid peptides. ENK, enkephalin; Dyn, dynorphin. Reproduced with permission from Akil et al. (1984) *Annual Review of Neuroscience* 7, 223–55.

second minor group of endorphin-containing neurones has recently been identified in the caudal part of the medulla. Enkephalins are much more widely distributed and are found in cell bodies and fibres throughout the brain. The dynorphin system is also widely distributed, but, as the diagrams in Fig. 5.2 show, the three opioid peptide families have distributions which do not completely overlap.

Dynorphins and endorphins are also found within the pituitary. In particular, dynorphins have been shown to coexist with ADH

Table 5.1. The amino acid sequences of a number of biologically active opioid peptides.

Beta-endorphin	Tyr−Gly−Gly−Phe−Met−Thr−Ser−Glu−Lys− Ser−Gln−Thr−Pro−Leu−Val−Thr−Leu−Phe− Lys−Asn−Ala−Ile−Val−Lys−Asn−Ala−His− Lys−Lys−Gly−Gln
Leu-enkephalin	Tyr−Gly−Gly−Phe−Leu
Met-enkephalin	Tyr−Gly−Gly−Phe−Met Tyr−Gly−Gly−Phe−Met−Arg−Phe Tyr−Gly−Gly−Phe−Met−Arg−Gly−Leu
Peptide E	Tyr−Gly−Gly−Phe−Met−Arg−Arg−Val−Gly− Arg−Pro−Glu−Trp−Trp−Met−Asp−Tyr−Gln− Lys−Arg−Tyr−Gly−Gly−Phe−Leu
Metorphamide	Tyr−Gly−Gly−Phe−Met−Arg−Arg−Val−NH_2
Amidorphan	Tyr−Gly−Gly−Phe−Met−Lys−Lys−Met−Asp− Glu−Leu−Tyr−Pro−Leu−Glu−Val−Glu−Glu− Glu−Ala−Asn−Gly−Gly−Glu−Val−Leu−NH_2
Dynorphin $_{1-17}$	Tyr−Gly−Gly−Phe−Leu−Arg−Arg−Ile−Arg− Pro−Lys−Leu−Lys−Trp−Asp−Asn−Gln
Dynorphin B	Tyr−Gly−Gly−Phe−Leu−Arg−Arg−Gln−Phe− Lys−Val−Val−Thr
Dynorphin $_{1-8}$	Tyr−Gly−Gly−Phe−Leu−Arg−Arg−Ile
Beta-neoendorphin	Tyr−Gly−Gly−Phe−Leu−Arg−Lys−Tyr−Pro
Alpha−neoendorphin	Tyr−Gly−Gly−Phe−Leu−Arg−Lys−Tyr−Pro− Lys

both in hypothalamic neurones and within the neural lobe. Endorphins, on the other hand, predominate in the anterior and intermediate lobes of the pituitary. There is as yet no clear physiological role for the minute amounts of endorphin-like immunoreactivity found in the peripheral circulation or the large amounts of enkephalins that are found in the peripheral nervous system (particularly in autonomic ganglia and within the adrenal medulla).

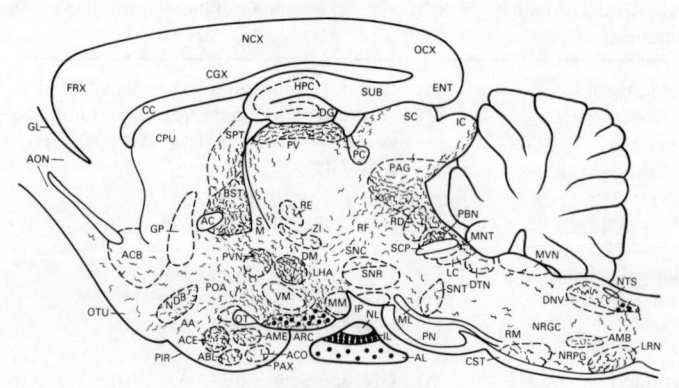

Chapter 5

Pro-opiomelanocortin

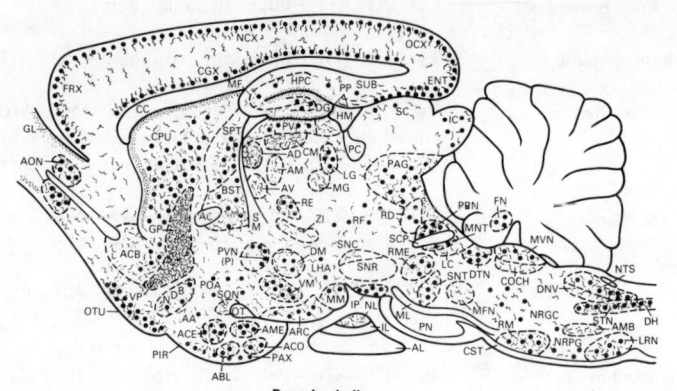

Proenkephalin

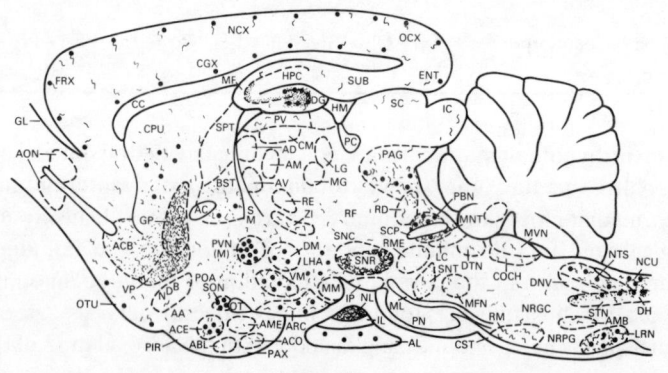

Prodynorphin

Fig. 5.2. Schematic representation of the distribution of pro-opiomelanocortin-, proenkephalin-, and prodynorphin-derived peptides in the rat CNS, as determined from immunohistochemical studies.

1 Pro-opiomelanocortin (POMC) contains one opioid peptide (β-endorphin), one copy of ACTH, and potentially three copies of MSH, namely α−, β−, and γ−MSH. In the brain, the major POMC neuronal population resides in the arcuate nucleus, with projections to many limbic and brainstem nuclei.

2 Proenkephalin codes for several peptides containing the opioid-active core Tyr−Gly−Gly−Phe−Met (or −Leu). These include one copy of [Leu]enkephalin, four copies of [Met]enkephalin−Arg−Phe and [Met]enkephalin−Arg−Gly−Leu. Peptides derived from proenkephalin are found in neuronal systems throughout the CNS, from the olfactory bulb to the spinal cord. These neurones form both local circuits and long-tract projections.

3 Prodynorphin also codes for several active opioid peptides containing the sequence of [Leu]enkephalin. These include dynorphin A, dynorphin B, and α-neoendorphin. This precursor is distributed in neuronal systems found at all levels of the neuraxis. Like their enkephalin counterparts, the prodynorphin neurones form both short- and long-tract projections — often found in parallel with the proenkephalin systems.

In these three parasagittal maps, neuronal cell bodies are shown as solid circles, and fibre terminals as short curved lines and dots. Each map represents multiple parasagittal levels through the rat brain and was reconstructed using the rat brain atlas of G. Paxinos and C. Watson (1982; *The Rat Brain in Stereotaxic Coordinates*. Academic Press, New York). Reproduced with permission from Khachaturian H., Lewis M.E., Schafer M.K.-H. & Watson S.J. (1985) *Trends in Neurosciences* **8**, 111−19. For key to abbreviations *see* original reference or Paxinos & Watson as above.

Opioid receptors

The first evidence for more than one type of opioid receptor came from clinical studies with nalorphine, which although it antagonizes the action of morphine can itself produce analgesia, together with other effects such as dysphoria and hallucinations. Martin *et al.* (1976) suggested that this substance could have a mixture of agonist and antagonist properties, such that it was an antagonist at the site at which morphine acted but an agonist at a second site. This suggestion led to a series of experiments in chronic spinal dogs in which the actions of a selection of natural and synthetic opioid drugs were found to differ in a number of pharmacological properties. As the drugs with which Martin worked were morphine, ketocyclazocine, and SKF 10047, he called the receptors mu, kappa, and sigma. The properties that were associated with each receptor are shown in Table 5.2.

Further evidence was soon forthcoming that there were indeed different types of opioid receptor. It was shown that isolated tissues such as the guinea pig ileum had a greater sensitivity to agents classified as kappa than did the mouse vas deferens, whereas these tissues were equally sensitive to mu agents. In contrast, the mouse vas deferens was much more sensitive to enkephalins than it was to mu agonists. On the guinea pig ileum the situation was reversed, so that normorphine was more active than the enkephalins. This led to the suggestion that a further opioid receptor existed, and this was called the delta receptor (from vas deferens). These four receptors (mu, delta, kappa, and sigma) have now been characterized in binding experiments using radiolabelled drugs. All are found to be present in mammalian brain (including that of man), and there are marked regional differences in the distribution of these receptors that can be visualized using the technique of autoradiography. There are also clear differences in the distribution and abundance of receptors between species, particularly for the kappa receptor. Man, for example, has a dense distribution of kappa receptors in many parts of the brain, whereas the rat is relatively deficient in kappa sites. The presence of different opioid receptor types on peripheral tissues helps to explain some of the unwanted side-effects of opioid drugs.

Table 5.2. Pharmacological actions of mu, kappa, and sigma agonists (after Martin).

	Mu	Kappa	Sigma
Pupil	Miosis	Miosis	Mydriasis
Respiratory rate	Depression	No change	Stimulation
Heart rate	Bradycardia	No change	Tachycardia
Behaviour	Indifference	Sedation	Delirium
Thermal pain	Analgesia	No effect	No effect
Mechanical pain	Analgesia	Analgesia	Weak analgesia

Pharmacology of Opioid Analgesics

The use of binding experiments, coupled with computer analysis of displacement curves, has allowed a detailed examination of the interaction of opioid drugs with the different receptor types. We now have very selective ligands for mu, delta, and kappa receptors that can be used as tools to identify new drugs acting at these sites, but most of the agents that are currently in clinical use are not particularly selective, and their observed actions are likely to be due to an action at more than one receptor. Examples of the receptor selectivity of a range of opioids are given in Table 5.3.

The functional role of each opioid receptor type is not easy to define. It is not possible to say, for instance, that one receptor is responsible for the production of analgesia, whereas the others are concerned with unwanted side-effects. Evidence currently available suggests that analgesia can be produced by activating mu, delta, or kappa receptors, but possibly not by activating sigma receptors. Some unwanted actions are associated with each receptor type, but they are sufficiently different to make it worthwhile to try to develop drugs that are selective for each receptor type.

Table 5.3. Receptor selectivity of opioid analgesics.

Drug	Receptor type			
	Mu	Kappa	Delta	Sigma
Morphine	A	a	a	x
Naloxone	Ant	Ant	Ant	x
Fentanyl	A	a	x	—
Pentazocine	pA	A	ant	A
Butorphanol	pA	A	Ant	A
Nalbuphine	Ant	pA	ant	a
Buprenorphine	pA	Ant	A	—
Meptazinol	ant(A)	—	A	—

Key: A, strong agonist; a, weak agonist; Ant, strong antagonist; ant, weak antagonist; pA, partial agonist; x, neglibible activity; —, no activity. These classifications are still open to debate, and in some cases information on the same drug obtained in different tests is contradictory e.g. the activity of meptazinol. The major sources used to compile the table are Hughes 1983; Hayes *et. al.* 1986: Sheehan *et. al.* 1986; Jackson & Sewell 1986.

The possible exception to this is the sigma receptor, which most would say is not a true opioid receptor at all but is more closely associated with the actions of drugs such as phencyclidine (PCP), which are powerfully psychotomimetic. Much work is currently in progress on sigma agents, chiefly due to their ability to interfere with excitatory amino acid-operated neurotransmission, and it is clear that there are likely to be subtypes of this receptor. Some further mention of sigma actions will be made in Chapter 6 when the analgesic properties of ketamine are considered, and a detailed discussion of the characteristics of drugs with actions at mu, delta, and kappa receptors will be given in later sections of this chapter.

The endogenous opioid peptides, in common with most other endogenous neural messengers, appear to be mixed agonists capable of acting at more than one opioid receptor type. A tentative assignment of receptor preference for the three peptide families is given in Table 5.4. The most interesting observation is that it is only the dynorphin family that has a distinct action at the kappa receptor.

Recently, suggestions have been made that there are further subtypes of opioid receptor, and, although in the long term this may be established unequivocally, the available evidence is not totally convincing. Pasternak (1980) and his colleagues have suggested that mu receptors can be divided into mu_1 and mu_2 variants on the basis of binding experiments with an antagonist called naloxazone. This substance blocks a binding site to which both morphine and enkephalins bind with high affinity (mu_1) and which is proposed to be the site responsible for analgesia. At a somewhat lower affinity site morphine binds with a higher affinity than enkephalins, and this is termed the mu_2 site. This classification has been used to explain the profile of the new analgesic meptazinol (on the basis that this is a selective mu_1 agonist) but this particular drug (of which more will be said later) has a rather

Table 5.4. Endogenous opioids: receptors at which they act.

Enkephalins	Delta>mu
Endorphins	Mu>delta
Dynorphins	Kappa>mu/delta

complicated action that includes non-opioid properties. Other postulated receptors (e.g. epsilon, lambda) are outside the scope of the present text.

Agonists, partial agonists, and antagonists

The result of a drug—receptor interaction depends on the site of the receptor and the type of receptor (e.g. activation of mu receptors in the periaqueductal grey matter will have different consequences to activating mu receptors in the myenteric plexus of the gut). It also depends upon the relative abundance of each receptor type at each site. The activity of opioid analgesics is further influenced by two factors, the selectivity of an individual drug for each particular receptor type, and the intrinsic activity at that receptor. Should a drug happen to be totally selective for one receptor type and also function as a full agonist at that site, then the situation is straightforward, but this is rarely encountered in practice.

A full agonist has a high intrinsic activity. This means that it can produce the maximum effect possible at the receptor type at which it acts by binding with a relatively small number of receptors. It is therefore active in tissues with a large population of receptors (high reserve) and in those with a small population (low reserve). In a situation where two drugs are given together the action of full agonists will be additive.

A partial agonist has a low intrinsic activity. In tissues with a high receptor reserve it produces a clear effect and is an agonist. In tissues with a low receptor reserve it occupies the receptors but produces no measurable effect. It therefore prevents the binding of an agonist and is an antagonist. Where an action is seen, this is likely to have a shallower dose—response curve than that for a full agonist under the same conditions, and a lower maximum response. Where two drugs are given together the interaction can be complex, but it is usually possible to demonstrate antagonism of the actions of a full agonist by a partial agonist.

A full antagonist such as naloxone will consistently antagonize the actions of both full and partial agonists without itself producing any agonist effects. It is possible for a drug to be a full agonist at one receptor and a partial agonist or antagonist at another. In binding experiments opioid drugs of all three types may have similar affinities, and it is therefore necessary to perform isolated smooth muscle experiments in order to characterize correctly the properties of a new agent. To this end it has been of great value to know that the guinea pig ileum has both mu and kappa receptors in high reserve, that the rabbit vas deferens has only kappa receptors in low reserve, and that the rat vas deferens has only mu receptors in low reserve. Some rather inadequate classification of agents as full or partial agonists has also been made on the basis of behavioural tests, and this is usually unreliable.

A number of drugs that have potent antagonist properties are now available and can be used to reverse the actions of opioids given in overdose. Agents that have a mixture of opioid agonist and antagonist action, e.g. nalorphine, do not have a role as antagonists in modern therapy, and their interactions in the patient can be complex. Those pure antagonists that are currently available are active at mu, delta and kappa receptors, although in general higher concentrations are needed for displacement from delta and kappa receptors. Naloxone is still the most widely used antagonist but has the disadvantages of a comparatively short duration of action (30—90 min depending on dose) and lack of oral bioavailability. Two newer but chemically related drugs, naltrexone and nalmefene, have advantages in both these areas. Quadazocine is an extremely potent antagonist at mu and kappa receptors that is currently under investigation.

Naloxone is free from side-effects until very high doses are reached when it will start to block GABA receptors. It is therefore proconvulsive and must be treated with caution in some situations (e.g. central excitation produced by large doses of pethidine).

Morphine

Morphine is the archetype opioid drug and will be used as a practical example of the pharmacological properties of drugs of this type. It is an agonist at the mu receptor and also has some kappa properties (*see* Table 5.3), although its affinity for mu sites is nearly 100 times greater. In most assays and in the clinical situation its mu properties predominate. It has little or no action at delta receptors and at sigma sites. Mechanisms for its analgesic action will be covered before dealing with its other actions. Possible sites of action are shown in Fig. 5.3.

Under some circumstances opioids may be able to produce analgesia by a peripheral mechanism, and like other peripherally acting analgesics they are then found to be more effective in the presence of inflammation. Studies by Smith *et al.* (1982) using *N*-methylmorphine as an agonist and *N*-methylnalorphine as an antagonist, because neither will significantly cross the blood—

Terminals   Axons   CNS

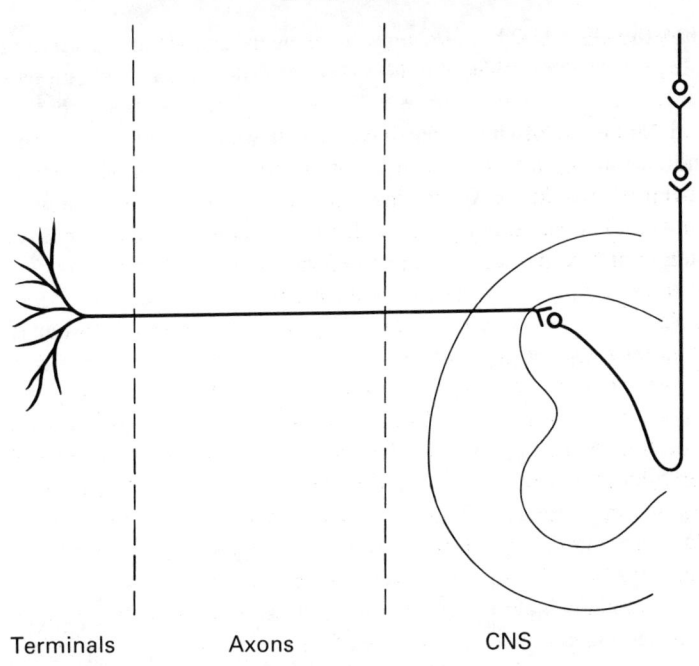

Fig. 5.3. From Hill *et al.* (1984) with permission.

brain barrier, have established this mechanism of action. Recently the same group have reported similar results using a polar enkephalin analogue, and is possible that a drug of this type may reach clinical use in the future.

The available evidence suggests that opioids stabilize the peripheral nerve terminals by reducing an inward calcium current (North & Egan 1983). The reduction in excitability of sensory nerve terminals resulting from this would be expected to raise the nociceptive threshold. It is not clear at present how much this type of action contributes to the therapeutic action of opioid analgesics. Opioids may also act on the axons transmitting nociceptive impulses into the central nervous system or on the sensory ganglia (*see* Fig. 5.3). Opioid binding has been detected on primary afferent fibres and on dorsal root ganglion cells, but it now seems that the peripheral parts of primary afferent fibres and dorsal root ganglion cells in mature animals are not sensitive to opioids and that the detected binding may have been to uncoupled binding sites rather than to functional receptors. This may reflect changes during development, as the cell bodies of dorsal root ganglion cells grown in tissue culture are sensitive to opioids. The third area for analgesic drug action is within the central nervous system. Although there is still some debate over the precise mechanisms of opioid analgesia, much experimental work has led to three suggestions which are summarized in diagrammatic form in Fig. 5.4. Although this is presented here in the context of the dorsal horn of the spinal cord, the same theoretical possibilities exist at ascending relays within the reticular formation and thalamus for example.

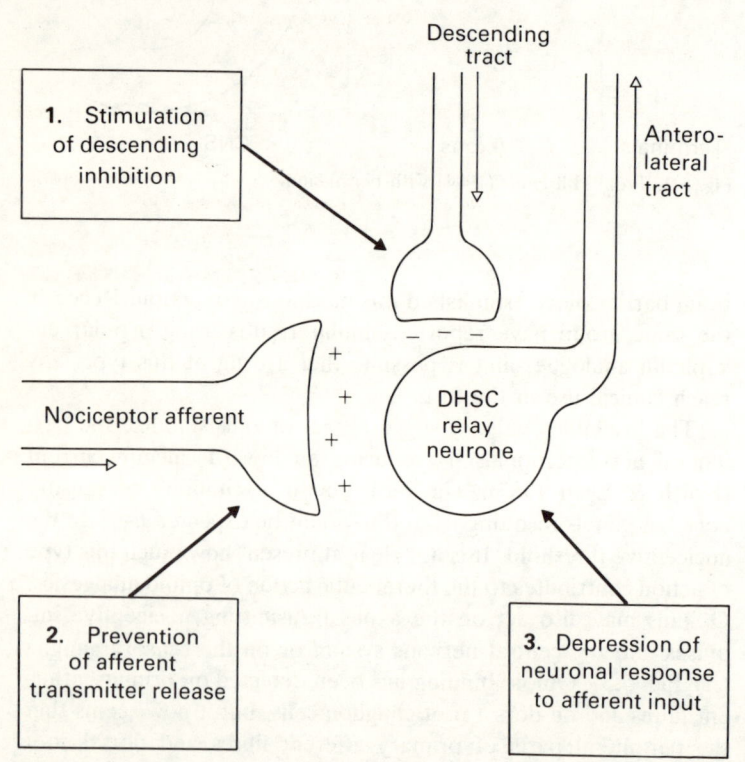

Fig. 5.4. From Hill *et al.* (1984) with permission.

1 *Stimulation of descending inhibition.* The concept of an opioid-stimulated descending inhibitory system arose from microinjection studies that revealed a region of great sensitivity adjacent to the third and fourth ventricles, where small doses of opioid would produce profound analgesia. Furthermore, it was found that behavioural analgesia produced by systemic administration of morphine could be attenuated by periaqueductal grey matter lesions or by injecting naloxone into this structure. It has been shown that nucleus raphe magnus stimulation will potentiate morphine analgesia in animals and that raphe lesions render morphine less effective. Morphine analgesia is attenuated but not abolished by lesions of the descending pathways within the posterolateral columns of the spinal cord (Basbaum *et al.* 1977).

2 *Prevention of primary afferent transmitter release.* When systemic opioids are administered whilst making microelectrode recordings from neurones in the dorsal horn of the spinal cord it is possible to show that the response to a peripheral noxious stimulus is blocked, leaving the response to non-noxious stimulation relatively unaffected (Duggan *et al.* 1976). When peripheral electrical stimuli are used to evoke the neuronal response the opioid effect can be seen to be a selective attenuation of the long latency response resulting from activation of C fibres, leaving the short latency response arriving in A fibres little affected (LeBars *et al.* 1976). Such selective effects are difficult to explain without suggesting that the opioids are acting on the presynaptic terminals of nociceptor fibres to inhibit transmitter release, but not on the larger non-nociceptive fibres. There is now evidence that opioids both *in vitro* and *in vivo* (Yaksh *et al.* 1980) will reduce the release of substance P and other excitatory peptides from unmyelinated primary afferents.

3 *Depression of neuronal response to afferent input.* Opioids have direct, postsynaptic effects on the firing of spinal and supraspinal neurones. This depression of neuronal firing is due to the opening of membrane potassium channels resulting in an outward current that hyperpolarizes the neurone and makes it less excitable (Williams *et al.* 1982). A minority of central neurones are excited by the application of opioids, but this effect is now thought to be due to inhibition of tonically active inhibitory interneurones and is

thus indirect (Henderson 1983). Part of the analgesic efficacy of opioids is therefore explicable by direct postsynaptic depression of neurones in nociceptive pathways. This depression has been reported on neurones at all levels between the spinal cord and the cerebral cortex, and it can therefore be seen that opioids will have multiple sites of action. It is unquestioned that there is an important spinal locus for opioid action, but some clinical observations would argue that supraspinal actions are at least as important (Wikler 1950). Thalamic nociceptive responses are much more sensitive to depression by intravenous morphine than are the nociceptive responses of spinal dorsal horn neurones (Hill *et al.* 1984). This high sensitivity can be explained quite easily, as polysynaptic responses are known to be more sensitive to depression by opioids (Jurna *et al.* 1973). In the clinical context a useful degree of analgesia may be obtained by actions at supraspinal sites with doses of morphine too small to produce a distinct effect at the spinal level.

The structure of morphine is shown in Fig. 5.5, together with the structure of fentanyl, which has a higher selectivity for the mu receptor than does morphine. Although at first sight there may not appear to be much resemblance between the two molecules, their pharmacological actions require that they are able to achieve similar conformations when in the immediate vicinity of the mu receptor so as to allow binding to take place. The required conformation is better illustrated by the molecule of morphine, which is rather rigid, than by the flexible fentanyl. Codeine, a commonly used weak opioid analgesic, is the methylether of morphine, and as it is virtually inactive *in vitro* it has been suggested that its *in*

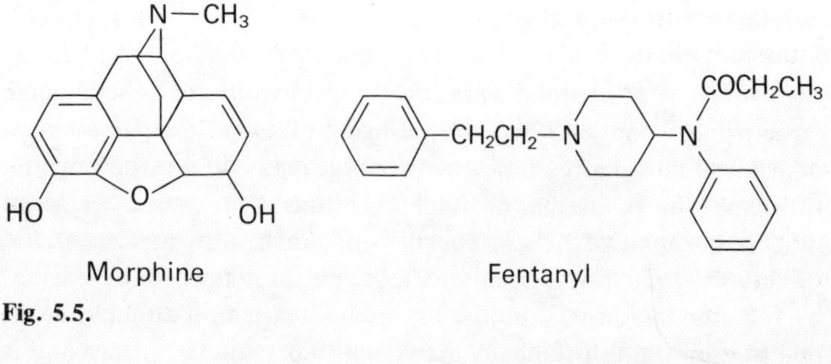

Morphine   Fentanyl

Fig. 5.5.

Pharmacology of Opioid Analgesics

vivo analgesic activity is solely due to the fact that it is metabolized to morphine.

All mu-selective opioid agonists are potent analgesics in a range of animal tests and in the clinic. They also tend to induce euphoria, and have a strong dependence liability, which, although not an impediment to use in postoperative pain, makes these drugs subject to legal controls which can make nursing staff in particular reluctant to agree to their use. Mu opioids are respiratory depressants and in high doses can be overtly sedative. They can produce nausea and vomiting and cause constipation.

The analgesic and side-effects all seem to be attributable to the same underlying mechanism of action whereby activation of receptors on the surface of neurones within the CNS or in the periphery leads to an increase in the outward movement of potassium ions. This in turn causes hyperpolarization of the cell membrane, thereby making the neurone less likely to fire an action potential. A similar mechanism is thought to operate on nerve terminals, where the increase in the outward potassium conductance leads indirectly to a decrease in the inward flow of calcium. This reduces transmitter release and impedes synaptic transmission. These actions within the central nervous system can produce analgesia, sedation, or euphoria, whereas when expressed on neurones within the gut will lead to constipation.

Mu opioids show reduced effectiveness if administered repeatedly at high doses, and this is usually referred to as tolerance. This phenomenon is not associated with a reduction in the number of opioid receptors present on the cell surface or with a change in the receptor binding characteristics. Although incompletely understood at present, it is probably due to an uncoupling of the cell surface receptors from the intracellular mechanism that opens the potassium channels. When prolonged high-dose administration of mu opioids is stopped then a withdrawal syndrome is seen, and this can also be precipitated without stopping the opioid if a potent antagonist drug such as naloxone is given. Typically withdrawal leads to sweating, cramps, diarrhoea, shivering, and general malaise, these symptoms being aborted if a large dose of mu agonist is given.

The practical use of morphine as an analgesic in postoperative pain is dealt with in Chapter 9.

Alternatives to morphine

Opioid drugs are classified according to the chemical series from which they are derived, but it should be noted that this can be unhelpful when their pharmacological profiles are considered, as drugs with very different properties can emerge from the same chemical series.

Papaveretum

This is a mixture of alkaloids extracted from opium. Its wanted and unwanted effects closely resemble those of morphine. It is difficult to justify the use of this mixture, rather than morphine alone, on pharmacological grounds. It contains 50% anhydrous morphine together with mainly papaverine, codeine, narcotine, and thebaine. It has been suggested that this preparation has an advantageous spectrum of action in colic, but it is unlikely that the amount of papaverine present would be large enough to have any significant antispasmodic effect. Twenty mg of papaveretum are equivalent to 12.5–13.1 mg of morphine sulphate.

Dihydromorphine (diamorphine, heroin)

This is the diacetyl derivative of morphine. There is some controversy over whether it is a more powerful analgesic than morphine, and it is probably of similar potency (no more than twice that of morphine) although its greater solubility allows larger doses to be administered in a given volume of injection, and it penetrates into the central nervous system more efficiently. In receptor binding experiments it is not possible to detect any affinity of heroin itself for mu receptors, although 6-acetylmorphine, one of its metabolites, is equipotent with morphine. The effect of a dose of dihydromorphine is in fact expressed as the effect of this substance and of morphine, which is also a metabolite. There is little point in using this drug rather than morphine in most therapeutic situations, although when used epidurally it has very different pharmacokinetics to morphine.

Codeine and dihydrocodeine

Codeine occurs naturally in opium, but that used clinically is made by the methylation of morphine. As mentioned above it is probable that codeine is only analgesic because of its hepatic metabolism to morphine. Dihydrocodeine is a synthetic compound with very similar properties, although it has been reported to produce a high incidence of hallucinations. Both these compounds are very much weaker analgesics than morphine. They are used alone, but increasingly drugs of this type are given in combination with a non-steroidal anti-inflammatory agent (*see later*).

Hydromorphone, oxycodone, and oxymorphone

These drugs are semisynthetic morphine derivatives with few if any advantages over their parent compound. Oxymorphone is available in the form of suppositories however, and can provide useful long-duration analgesia when used by that route.

Levorphanol and phenazocine

These are synthetic morphine analogues (morphinans) whose pharmacology is not significantly different to that of morphine. Levorphanol is the one that has received most clinical use. The view found in some textbooks that it produces analgesia without sedation has no pharmacological rationale, and has been disputed in the clinical literature. It has a faster onset of action than morphine and a longer duration of action (8–14 hours). It has a higher oral bioavailability than most other opioids, but it has been reported to give variable responses in different patients, and this has probably limited its use. Phenazocine has also been claimed to have little sedative action but not all reports agree on this. It is active sublingually and causes less increase in biliary pressure than most opioids.

Pethidine

This is a totally synthetic compound that has a similar receptor binding profile to morphine, being largely mu-selective, although it may have slightly more kappa properties than morphine. It has a much higher lipophilicity than morphine, and more of a given dose will reach the central nervous system. In addition to the opioid properties shared with morphine, pethidine has atropine-like actions, which according to the clinical context may be advantageous or not. It can cause severe depression of the cardiovascular system in overdose, and its principal metabolite, norpethidine, is a convulsant that can also cause hallucinations in lower doses. Naloxone may exacerbate the convulsions produced as a result of pethidine overdose. It is more locally irritant to the tissues than morphine, but has better oral bioavailability. Constipation and urinary retention are less common with pethidine, and it causes less spasm of the biliary tract. It is a mild stimulant of uterine contraction (cf. the antioxytocic action of morphine, fentanyl, etc.), and it appears to cause less respiratory depression of the newborn than either morphine or methadone. Its continued use may be more historical (due to its unsupervised use by midwives) than logical, and although it may be possible to argue that it has advantages over morphine for obstetric use it is difficult to establish a role for it as an agent of choice in the treatment of postoperative pain.

Fentanyl, alfentanil and sufentanil

These compounds are all potent mu-selective agents and are chemically very closely related to each other and to pethidine. Fentanyl is some 50–100 times more potent than morphine as an analgesic, but a large part of this difference is due to increased lipophilicity rather than to increased affinity for the mu receptor. It has a short duration of action that limits its general utility. Alfentanil is similar to fentanyl but it has a more rapid onset and even shorter duration of action. Sufentanil is probably the most selective non-peptide ligand for the mu receptor yet available. In man it has been claimed to have 600 times the analgesic potency of morphine. It again has a short duration of action, which will probably limit its use.

Fentanyl is not generally used for postoperative pain, as doses which do not cause ventilatory depression have a short duration of action. However, larger doses used as part of the anaesthetic sequence may remain active well into the postoperative period. The increased popularity of patient-controlled analgesia and intravenous and epidural infusions is associated with an increased use of fentanyl. It appears to cause less sedation than morphine, but high doses and/or prolonged use may lead to muscular rigidity.

It has a number of pathways for biotransformation and elimination, and as its metabolites are inactive it is useful in hepatic and renal disease. A new long-acting analogue, lofentanil, shows promise as a spinally administered opioid.

Phenoperidine, anileridine, and alphaprodine

These are all relatives of pethidine with very similar properties.

Methadone

This is a totally synthetic opioid of the diphenylpropylamine class. Its pharmacology is broadly similar to that of morphine and it is mu-selective. It has a very much longer plasma half-life than morphine, and this is reflected in a longer duration of action. It tends to accumulate in the body on repeated administration, particularly in elderly patients. In the immediate postoperative period the duration of useful analgesia is 6–8 hours after a 10 mg dose, but continued or repeated use causes prolonged or accentuated effects. Its slow onset and offset of action make it less liable to abuse than other mu opioids. It has no effect on the uterus and is effective orally.

Dipipanone and dextromoramide

These are chemical analogues of methadone with similar pharmacology. They have few if any therapeutic advantages. Some clinical studies show that dextromoramide produces a shorter period of analgesia (2–3 hours) than would be predicted by the plasma half-life of the drug, and this probably reflects the lack of persistence of active drug within the central nervous system.

Dextropropoxyphene

This is a weak analgesic of the same chemical class as methadone. It has good oral bioavailability and approximately the same order of potency as codeine, and has similar side-effects. In common with other weak opioids it is most frequently used in combination with paracetamol.

Agents with a mixture of agonist and antagonist properties

Buprenorphine

Buprenorphine is an oripavine derivative of thebaine and is chemically similar to etorphine, an extremely potent opioid used to immobilize big game animals. It is therefore not surprising that it produces analgesia in man with doses as low as 2−4 µg/kg. The pharmacology of buprenorphine is complex, but it is best classified as a high-affinity partial agonist at the mu receptor and a kappa antagonist. It has a higher delta affinity than most non-peptide opioids. The abuse liability appears to be low, although it will suppress morphine withdrawal symptoms. It is not orally bioavailable as it is metabolized by gut wall enzymes, but it is effective when given by injection or sublingually. It has a long duration of action.

Effective analgesia can be obtained in most patients with this drug in spite of its partial agonist character, and it can also cause ventilatory depression. It is not easily displaced from the opioid receptor, and therefore its action is not reliably reversed by naloxone. Ventilatory depression may need to be treated with stimulants such as doxapram or with ventilatory support. It may be difficult to achieve analgesia with opioids in a patient who is receiving, without effect, high doses of buprenorphine.

Pentazocine

This was the first compound available for use in man with significant agonist activity at the kappa receptor. It is an antagonist at mu receptors and also has a high affinity for sigma sites (probably explaining its ability to produce hallucinations). It is well absorbed from injection sites but its oral bioavailability is poor (<20%). It has a lower maximum analgesic effect than morphine, and increasing the dose in an attempt to increase the analgesic effect (i.e. above 40 mg) leads to an escalation of side-effects, which include nausea, dizziness, sedation, and hallucinations (which are more vivid and unpleasant than those produced by morphine or pethidine). It increases the systemic and pulmonary arterial pressures and increases cardiac work. Like pethidine it increases uterine contractility, but it passes through the placental barrier less readily.

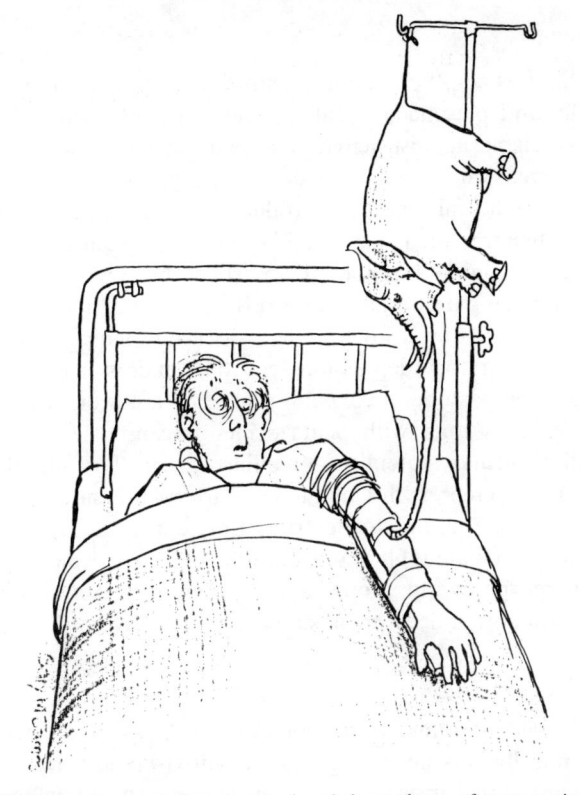

Hallucinations may be associated with large doses of pentazocine.

Nalbuphine

This is a recently introduced semisynthetic opioid drug that is similar in properties to pentazocine. It is a partial agonist at kappa receptors and a mu antagonist. Although it has sigma affinity, this property is less apparent than in pentazocine. Its mu actions are complex, as in some situations it can suppress morphine withdrawal symptoms, suggesting that it might have partial agonist activity. It is well absorbed following intramuscular injection and has about 25% oral bioavailability.

This drug does not increase pulmonary artery pressure or cardiac work. The maximum analgesic effect is reached at a dose of 30 mg, and it appears to be relatively safe despite isolated reports of delayed cardiorespiratory depression (Lawrie & Drake 1985).

Butorphanol

Butorphanol is another recently introduced opioid. It is both chemically and pharmacologically related to pentazocine. It has kappa and sigma agonist activity and is a mu partial agonist (or possibly a weak full agonist). It does not suppress or precipitate morphine withdrawal, but it can produce a strong abstinence reaction itself when treatment is stopped (which argues against it being a simple kappa agonist). It is not well absorbed when given orally and even when given parenterally its short duration of action (90 min) limits its utility. It has a low ceiling to its action which limits the amount of respiratory depression seen but renders it ineffective against severe postoperative pain. There is a lower frequency of hallucinations than with pentazocine. It causes less nausea, constipation, urinary retention, or biliary spasm than morphine. Butorphanol increases the pulmonary artery pressure but decreases heart rate and systemic arterial pressure.

Pentazocine, nalbuphine and butorphanol are all more sedative than morphine (in proportion to their analgesic potency), and this probably reflects their kappa agonist activity.

Meptazinol

This is a drug with a mixture of opioid and non-opioid properties. It is chemically unique, being a hexahydroazepine, and it has been suggested that it owes much of its action to being an agonist for the mu_1 receptor. It behaves as a mu antagonist in as much as it will precipitate withdrawal in morphine-dependent animals. It has cholinomimetic properties that contribute to its analgesic action. Although naloxone will reverse most of its actions, hyoscine is needed for complete reversal. It has little respiratory depressant action in low doses, but large doses will cause this. It is well absorbed after intramuscular injection, but oral absorption is poor. Side-effects have been reported to limit its use, and emesis is particularly prevalent. It can be metabolized by the neonate and has been compared favourably with pethidine for obstetric use.

Dezocine

This is another chemically novel agent (an aminotetralin) that has weak kappa agonist properties and strong mu antagonist actions. It does not substitute for morphine in dependent animals

Pharmacology of Opioid Analgesics

but will precipitate withdrawal. It is therefore paradoxical that addicts will describe dezocine as morphine-like when it is administered under blind conditions. It actions seem to be only partially reversible with naloxone and it can cause severe respiratory depression. Clinical experience with this agent is limited.

New developments

Most of the research effort invested in new opioid analgesics is in order to avoid the unwanted effects of mu opioids (Table 5.5.), and considerable progress has been made in the shape of selective kappa agonists that have little or no action at other opioid receptors. The structures of a range of kappa agonists are shown in Fig. 5.6. The archetype kappa agonist is ethylketocyclazocine (EKC), but although this is a highly potent kappa agonist it is also a mu partial agonist is and has strong sigma actions. Bremazocine and tifluadom are more recently developed agents that also combine powerful kappa agonism with action at other opioid receptors. The first adequately selective kappa agonist to be available for detailed study was the Upjohn compound, U50488. This has a kappa affinity 80-fold higher than its mu affinity and has negligible action at sigma or delta sites. A later relative of this drug, called U69593, is similar in most respects but has a 300-fold separation between its kappa and mu actions, and a third compound, U62066 (spiradoline), is currently on clinical trial. When the results of these studies are available it will be possible, for the first time, to make an objective assessment of the likely clinical utility of a selective kappa agonist. Various clues as to the range of actions expected are already available from studies with less selective agents, and the probable advantages and disadvantages of kappa agonists are summarized in Table 5.6.

Table 5.5. Mu analgesics: limiting side-effects.

1 Constipation
2 Nausea/vomiting and dysphoria
3 Respiratory depression
4 Dependence liability
5 Sedation

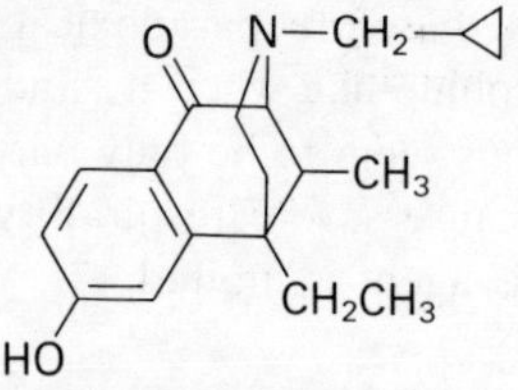

Ethylketocyclazocine

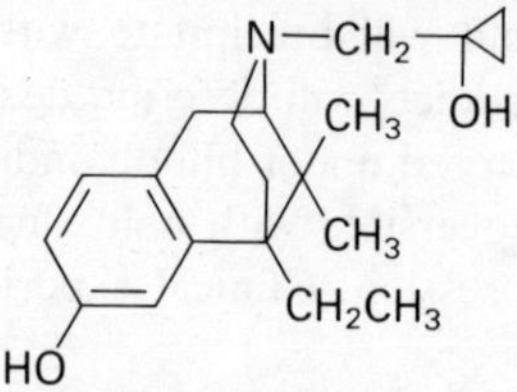

Bremazocine

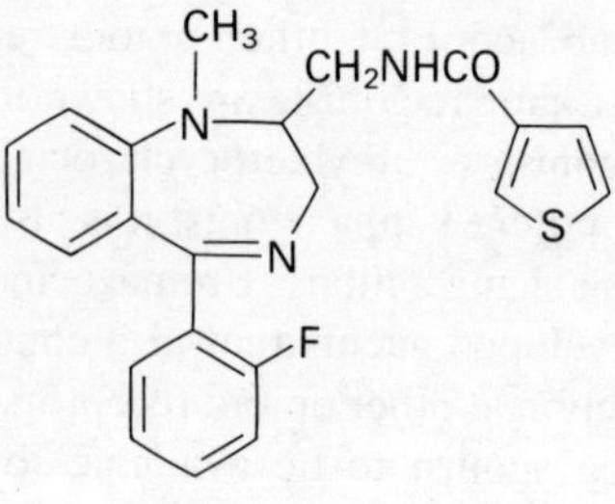

Tifluadom

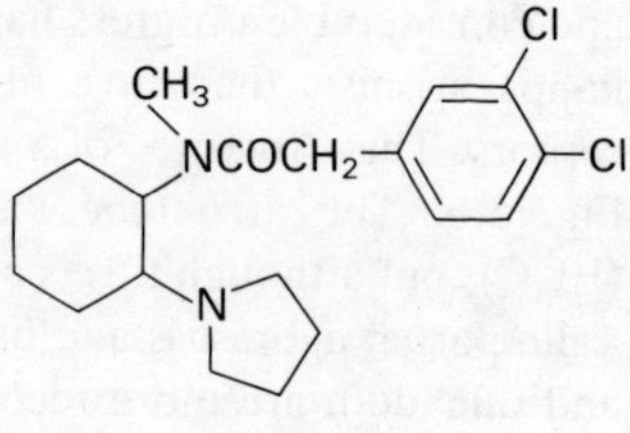

U50488

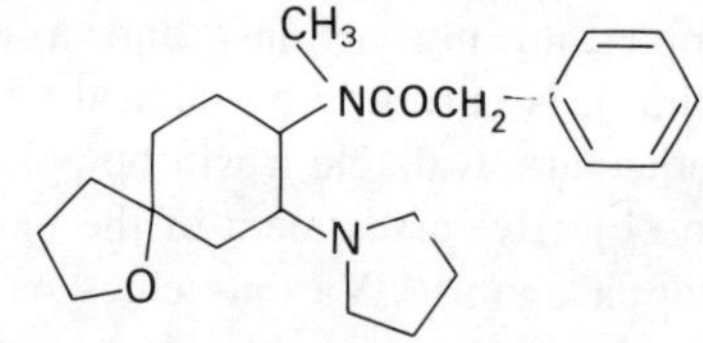

U69593

Fig. 5.6.

The problem of the sedative action of kappa agonists that has already been mentioned in relation to pentazocine can possibly be avoided by using a high-affinity kappa partial agonist rather than a full agonist. Xorphanol, a compound with kappa partial agonist and mu antagonist actions, is much less sedative than full kappa agonists such as U50488 when they are compared in animal tests, yet is an effective analgesic. This has been explained (Tyers *et al.*

Pharmacology of Opioid Analgesics

Table 5.6. Kappa analgesics.

Advantages	Disadvantages
1 Low abuse potential	1 Sedative
2 Non-constipating	2 Diuretic
3 No respiratory depression	3 ?Psychotomimetic
4 Powerful analgesia	4 ?Appetite stimulant

1986) in terms of there being a high receptor reserve in the parts of the brain where xorphanol acts to produce analgesia but a low receptor reserve in the area responsible for sedation. It will not be possible to validate this hypothesis until we have a kappa partial agonist without actions at other opioid receptors.

Recently another opioid strategy for producing analgesia has arisen with the observation that peptides selective for delta receptors produce analgesia when injected centrally in rats and mice. The delta-specificity of these results was confirmed using the delta-selective antagonist ICI 174864 (Rodriguez *et al.* 1986). There are not as yet delta-selective non-peptide opioids available for clinical evaluation, but experiments with spinal administration of available delta agonist peptides in terminal cancer patients showed that excellent analgesia could be produced when tolerance to the effects of morphine was evident (Yaksh *et al.* 1986). We now know that activation of mu and delta receptors turns on a common intracellular messenger system so that the physiological consequences are likely to be similar. It is therefore possible that delta agonists will share most if not all of the disadvantages of mu agonists. Kappa agonists, on the other hand, seem to have a distinct and different mechanism and therefore will have a very different range of actions.

CHAPTER 6
The Pharmacology of Non-Opioid Analgesics

Cyclo-oxygenase inhibitors and related drugs

As outlined in Chapter 2, pain may most commonly be produced as a result of tissue damage which causes release of pain-producing substances (algogens), which in turn excite the peripheral terminals of nociceptive afferent fibres. This action of algogens is potentiated by prostanoids, which are also produced in damaged tissue. Disruption of cell membranes causes release of phospholipids, which are acted on by phospholipase to produce arachidonic acid. This process can be inhibited by glucocorticosteroids. The prostanoids arise as a result of the action of cyclo-oxygenase on arachidonic acid to produce unstable cyclic endoperoxide intermediates, which break down to give prostacyclin, stable prostaglandins such as PGE_2, and thromboxanes. The most abundant prostanoid produced in inflamed tissues appears to be prostaglandin E_2, although thromboxanes and prostacyclin can also be detected. A second pathway of arachidonic acid metabolism, which may also be operational in damaged tissues, produces leukotrienes via the enzyme lipoxygenase. It is uncertain at present whether leukotrienes have any direct action on the activation of nociceptors. The process of arachidonic acid metabolism is summarized in Fig. 6.1.

In human pharmacological studies it has been determined that application of PGE_2 to a blister base does not itself cause pain, but interestingly tissue made oedematous by intradermal PGE injection becomes hyperalgesic. Following the original observation by Ferreira in 1972 that in man the pain response to intradermal bradykinin or histamine was much enhanced by simultaneous injection of PGE_1, potentiation of algogens with prostaglandins has been shown in a variety of preparations and species. The interaction with bradykinin is particularly strong, and bradykinin is well known to stimulate the production of prostaglandins, making it likely that these substances interact following their liberation

```
                    Tissue damage
                          │
                          │  Phospholipase   ┌─────────┐
                          │                  │ Steroids │
                          │                  └─────────┘
                          ▼
                    Arachidonic acid
         ┌─────────────┐ ╱           ╲  ┌──────────┐
         │   NSAIDs    │╱             ╲ │ BW 755C  │
         │ (e.g. aspirin)│             ╲│          │
         └─────────────┘╲               └──────────┘
                    Cyclo-oxygenase   Lipoxygenase
                          ▼                   ▼
              (Cyclic endoperoxides)      Leukotrienes
               ╱         │        ╲
              ╱          │         ╲
             ▼           ▼          ▼
        Thromboxanes  Prostacyclin  Stable
                                    prostaglandins
```

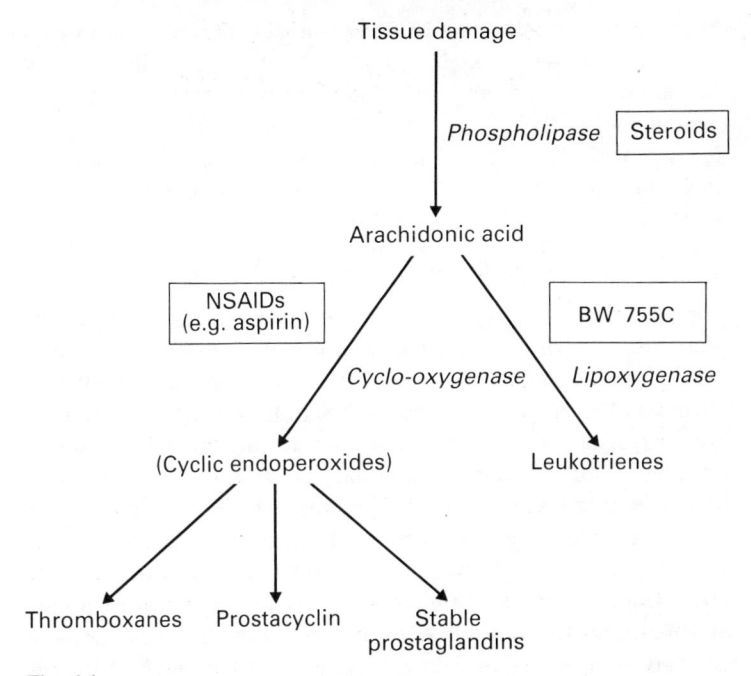

Fig. 6.1.

in damaged tissues. Non-steroidal anti-inflammatory drugs such as aspirin will not block the activation of nociceptors produced by combined injections of prostaglandins and algogens, as NSAIDs have no action on these receptors. When pain is intensified by the production of prostaglandins in damaged tissues, drugs such as aspirin can produce pain relief by blocking the action of cyclo-oxygenase, thereby inhibiting the synthesis of prostaglandins. Although, as mentioned above and in Fig. 6.1, the significance of leukotrienes in pain production is not understood at present, there are drugs in development that inhibit both cyclo-oxygenase and lipoxygenase (dual inhibitors, e.g. BW 755C), and it is possible that an agent of this type might ultimately prove to be a superior analgesic.

Drugs that are currently in clinical use and that probably owe their clinical utility to inhibition of cyclo-oxygenase include aspirin, ibuprofen, naproxen, fenbufen, diflunisal, piroxicam, indomethacin, and diclofenac. Individual agents, together with their relative advantages and disadvantages for use in postoperative pain are discussed in Chapter 9. They have, however, a number of common unwanted side-effects that are probably a consequence of their action on cyclo-oxygenase. The most important is probably damage to the gastric mucosa caused by removal of the prostaglandins that normally exert a cytoprotective action. 'Aspirin asthma' is also a fairly common side-effect, and although sometimes due to a true allergic reaction it may also be caused by the blockade of cyclo-oxygenase. This leads to the enhancement of production of lipoxygenase products such as the leukotrienes (e.g. SRS-A) which can directly cause bronchoconstriction and damage to the gastric mucosa. There is a school of thought that attributes the analgesic action of NSAIDs to factors other than cyclo-oxygenase inhibition, and it is interesting that three recently introduced drugs, etodolac, ketorolac, and anirolac, have analgesic potencies that are far higher than would be suggested by their abilities to inhibit cyclo-oxygenase. Ketorolac, in particular, was claimed to be as effective as morphine in the treatment of postoperative pain when both were given orally in a dose of 10 mg. When given intravenously, doses of 30 and 90 mg of ketorolac were claimed to be the equivalent of 12 mg of morphine given by this route. Analgesia lasted for 5–6 hours (compared to three hours with morphine) and side-effects were minor. These drugs clearly have potential value in the control of postoperative pain.

Centrally acting cyclo-oxygenase inhibitors

Paracetamol is something of an anomaly, as it has little if any anti-inflammatory action but is an effective analgesic. This has been explained by its ability to block the cyclo-oxygenase found within the central nervous system but not that found in peripheral tissues. This implies a role for prostanoids in the central end of the pain perception process, and it has been experimentally observed that injection of prostaglandin E_2 into the cerebral ventricles of a rat would potentiate the hyperalgesic effect of peripheral injection of this substance. It has been suggested that release of prostaglandins within the CNS might 'lower the threshold of the central pain circuits'.

Recently Sterling–Winthrop has revealed that it has an orally and parenterally active analgesic, Win-48098-6, that will inhibit

CNS cyclo-oxygenase. It is effective against types of experimental pain in animals (e.g. thermal) that are sensitive to morphine but not to NSAIDs such as aspirin. It is non-sedative and has no tendency to produce gastric or intestinal irritation and/or ulceration in rats as it does not inhibit peripheral cyclo-oxygenase. At present it is in clinical trial against postoperative pain, and it may prove to be an effective analgesic with few side-effects.

Nitrous oxide

It has been known for many years that nitrous oxide has useful analgesic properties when used in subanaesthetic doses, and its practical application is discussed in a later chapter. The mode of action of nitrous oxide appears to be markedly different to that of other inhalational anaesthetics. In some respects the analgesia produced by nitrous oxide resembles that produced by morphine. There is evidence from animal studies and in man that nitrous oxide analgesia can be reversed by opioid antagonists such as naloxone. Its analgesic effect is reduced in animals made tolerant to morphine. It is unlikely that a simple molecule such as that of nitrous oxide binds directly to opioid receptors, and therefore the probability is that it releases endogenous opioids within the brain. Support for this hypothesis comes from the observation that nitrous oxide will increase circulating levels of endorphin-like immunoreactivity (ELI) in women in labour. This release does not achieve levels sufficient to have analgesic effect *per se*, and its origin is the pituitary rather than brain, but if a similar release process occurs from neurones within the CNS it might well lead to the production of analgesia.

Ketamine

Ketamine is a derivative of phencylidine (PCP, a major hallucinogenic drug of abuse) and shares many of its properties. In high doses ketamine is an anaesthetic, but subanaesthetic doses are strongly analgesic. Practical aspects of the use of this substance in postoperative pain are dealt with later, but it should be noted that it has a complex pharmacology in addition to its analgesic actions.

Central effects include vivid dreams that may be unpleasant, and sometimes hallucinations (emergence reaction). The mechanism for these actions may or may not be related to the mechanism that is responsible for the analgesic effects of the drug. This is its ability to bind to the so-called sigma opioid receptor (now generally called the PCP receptor), a property shared with a number of opioid drugs, including SKF 10047 and pentazocine. There is also a second sigma site that has been characterized as a high-affinity binding site that ketamine and PCP do not compete for but from which labelled SKF 10047 can be displaced by haloperidol. The functional significance of this second sigma site is not completely clear at the present time.

The PCP site is intimately associated with one of the excitatory amino acid receptors that has been defined by its activation by a synthetic amino acid, *N*-methyl-D-aspartate (NMDA), and it is therefore referred to as the NMDA receptor. This receptor is used in synaptic transmission between different areas of the central nervous system, particularly in sensory systems, but probably not at the first synapse within the dorsal horn of the spinal cord. The analgesic properties of ketamine may be due to a reduction in nociceptive information traffic in ascending excitatory amino acid pathways linking spinal cord, brainstem, and thalamus. Hallucinatory and perceptual distortion effects could be produced by similar actions in visual and low-threshold somatic pathways. There is no direct competition between the binding of ketamine or PCP and that of excitatory amino acids, but the PCP binding site seems to be linked to the receptor complex beyond the recognition site (perhaps to the ion channel, as at other sites PCP is known to function as a channel blocker) (Fig. 6.2). Opioid drugs such as pentazocine which have a high affinity for the PCP/sigma site probably exert most of their analgesic action via classical opioid receptors, but have a psychotomimetic action by virtue of their sigma affinity.

Ketamine also has significant cardiovascular actions that are probably related to its ability to interact with ion channels rather than with the NMDA receptor. It can produce an increase in blood pressure and heart rate, and this has been suggested to be due to an increase in inward Ca^{2+} flux in cardiac muscle. Sympathetic reflexes are also blocked, possibly as a consequence of its action on sensory neurotransmission.

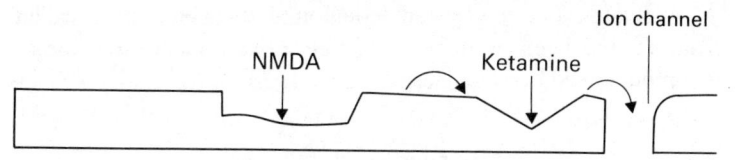

Fig. 6.2. Ketamine may bind within the ion channel or to an adjacent site (as shown here) within the NMDA receptor complex.

Nefopam

This is a unique drug that is structurally related to the antihistamine diphenhydramine, although it does not have any antihistamine properties itself. In animal tests for analgesic activity this agent is very weak, but it appears to have significant analgesic activity in man. Its mode of action is not fully understood, but is central rather than peripheral and is non-opioid. It excites reticular formation neurones at the origin of descending inhibitory pathways to the spinal cord, and this is probably due to monoamine release or its reported ability to block monoamine uptake.

There is some controversy over its use as a clinical analgesic, but there is more general agreement about its wide variety of unwanted actions, which include anxiety, restlessness, sweating, and nausea (possibly due to activation of monoamine systems in the CNS). It has weak anticholinergic properties that can produce dryness of the mouth and blurred vision (and which are exacerbated by its central sympathomimetic action).

Alpha$_2$ receptor agonists

The alpha$_2$ agonist clonidine, which is better known for its cardiovascular actions, is a powerful analgesic in a variety of animal tests. This action is accompanied by marked sedation, and both effects are likely to be due to depression of neuronal activity which is a consequence of activation of postsynaptic alpha$_2$ receptors, leading to activation of an outward potassium conductance. This is very similar to the final common pathway for the action of mu and delta opioids (*see* Chapter 5) and is likely to be the mechanism by which clonidine is able to suppress opioid withdrawal symptoms in dependent individuals, although clonidine does not interact directly with opioid receptors. Subthreshold doses of clonidine and morphine have an additive analgesic action.

A related but less potent compound than clonidine, called xylazine, has been used for some time in veterinary medicine as a combined sedative/analgesic.

Flupirtine and tazadolene

Flupirtine is a centrally acting analgesic of unknown mechanism of action. It produces analgesia in man after oral or rectal administration. Peak effect is reached in 30 min and analgesia lasts 3–5 hours. In a double-blind trial it was found that 100 mg of flupirtine had the effectiveness of 1 g of paracetamol or of 50 mg of pentazocine. Its chief advantage appears to be freedom from side-effects. Tazadolene is another non-opioid, centrally acting analgesic that is currently on clinical trial. It has antidepressant properties in addition to its analgesic properties. No data on clinical effectiveness have yet been published, but it is thought to be analgesic in man.

Bradykinin antagonists

Bradykinin is the most potent pain-producing substance (algogen) known to be released following tissue damage in man. It also produces release of substances which will potentiate its own action, and that of the prostaglandins and vasoactive peptides such as substance P. It will also potentiate the pain-producing action of other products of tissue damage such as 5-hydroxytryptamine. It can thus be considered as being the trigger for a complex process that will result in the production of pain. Recent work has identified two receptors for bradykinin, which are termed B_1 and B_2. It is the B_2 type that appears to be located on nociceptive afferent terminals, and a number of synthetic peptide analogues of bradykinin will antagonize its action at these receptors. These antagonists have been shown in man to block the pain produced by topical bradykinin, but not that produced by other algogens. It has been proposed that the pain due to, for example, burns could be treated with an aerosol containing a peptide bradykinin antagonist. This is likely to be a very limited form of therapy, although possibly worth trying as a topical application to an operative site. General use of bradykinin antagonists as analgesics must await the development of a stable (almost certainly nonpeptide) molecule that could be administered parenterally or orally.

CHAPTER 7
The Pharmacology of Drugs with Secondary Analgesic Properties

Many drugs which can be used in the production of analgesia are not analgesic in themselves but are of benefit by, for example, relieving an associated depressed state. Some have analgesic properties but are usually prescribed for some other indication. The collection of therapeutic agents considered here is not exhaustive, but all have been found to be of benefit in a number of distinct conditions (but not always to date in postoperative pain). A useful review of some of the issues was written by Budd (1981).

Anticonvulsants

Carbamazepine is an anticonvulsant that is well known to be of benefit in the treatment of the pain of trigeminal neuralgia. It has also been found of benefit in some patients with diabetic and uraemic peripheral neuropathies. Rapeport *et al.* (1984) found significant dose-related pain relief in a group of patients with peripheral nerve injuries or post-herpetic neuralgia treated with carbamazepine. Phenytoin and sodium valproate have also been found to be of value in some patients suffering pain of a paroxysmal, stabbing character. These three anticonvulsants have a common mode of action in that they bind to the inactive state of the neuronal sodium channel. As a consequence, when the neurone fires rapidly an increasing number of sodium channels become trapped in their inactive state. Hyperpolarization of the neurone allows the drug to leave the channel so that its ability to function is restored. The functional consequence of this type of action is that the transmission of a single impulse by nerves is little affected, but paroxysmal trains of impulses soon decay. Doses of valproate and phenytoin that are higher than those needed to attenuate repetitive firing potentiate the action of the inhibitory neurotransmitter gamma-aminobutyric acid (GABA) and this action may also contribute to analgesia (*see below* under Benzodiazepines).

Monoamine uptake blockers

The tricyclic antidepressants such as imipramine and amitriptyline block the re-uptake of monoamines into presynaptic terminals of central nervous system neurones. This has the effect of increasing the concentration of active amine at the synapse and maintaining that concentration for an extended period of time . In the context of analgesia it is the ability to enhance the action of 5-hydroxytryptamine-utilizing pathways that is of most significance. As discussed in Chapter 5, part of the action of morphine-like narcotic analgesics is expressed through descending monoamine pathways exerting an inhibitory influence on the dorsal horn of the spinal cord, and it is therefore not surprising that uptake blockers will potentiate the analgesic action of opioids. It should be noted, however, that drug metabolism interactions also occur, and some tricyclics will raise plasma morphine concentrations by competing for hepatic metabolizing enzymes. It is now accepted that in some patients, perhaps those who achieve the higher plasma levels of the drug (*see* Edelbroek *et al.* 1986), there is an acceptable level of analgesia produced by a tricyclic antidepressants alone. The correlation between pain and depression should not be neglected, and persistent pain may well need therapy for both conditions, although this should not be a common scenario with postoperative pain.

Monoamine oxidase inhibitors

This class of drug prevents breakdown of monoamine neurotransmitters by the enzyme monoamine oxidase, and thus is in some ways analogous to the uptake blockers. It is clear that in the treatment of pain their actions differ, and monoamine oxidase inhibitors have been found most useful in atypical pains where other agents have failed to produce relief. Phenelzine and tranylcypromine have been used in this context, but their use is severely limited by the delayed onset of action and the need to guard against adverse reactions caused by monoamines contained in food or other medication taken at the same time.

Amphetamine and cocaine

Prior to the introduction of strict controls on amphetamine because of its abuse potential, it was not uncommon to find it included in compound analgesic formulations. Recently interest in the ability of amphetamine to potentiate morphine has revived, and in one clinical study on postoperative pain it was found that 10 mg of dextroamphetamine would double the analgesic effect of a dose of morphine given at the same time (Forrest et al. 1977). It was noted, however, that the incidence of side-effects was somewhat higher than with morphine alone. The reasons for this action of amphetamine are complex and likely to be due to its ability to release catecholamines from stores within central nervous system terminals and to block monoamine uptake, and by an agonist action at 5-hydroxytryptamine receptors. Higher doses of amphetamine will also block monoamine oxidase. It should be remembered that parenteral administration of amphetamine in man is likely to lead to sympathomimetic effects such as tachycardia, and there may be a sharp rise in blood pressure.

Cocaine has also been coadministered with morphine and heroin, most commonly as the well-known Brompton Cocktail (which was first used in the treatment of postoperative pain following thoracotomy). It was believed that cocaine would enhance the analgesia produced by the opioids, but in an objective trial of the analgesic effects of morphine or heroin with or without cocaine Twycross (1979) found that cocaine had no effect on the patients' perception of their pain. There is also uncertainty over whether there is any useful increase in alertness when cocaine is added to opioids, and as some patients become agitated and hallucinate on such mixtures there seems to be a strong argument for using opioids alone. On theoretical grounds cocaine should be able to duplicate most of the effects produced by amphetamine, as it blocks the re-uptake of noradrenaline into nerve terminals and thereby potentiates noradrenergic transmission. Recent experiments in rats have shown that morphine analgesia can be potentiated by cocaine, and that this is likely to be a result of blockade of noradrenaline uptake (Misra et al. 1987). It does not, however, act as an agonist at 5HT receptors (and indeed may well be an antagonist at $5HT_3$ sites). As it is this property of amphetamine that is most likely to lead to the potentiation of morphine analgesia, it may explain the differences between these two agents.

Phenothiazines and butyrophenones

This group of drugs, although best known as antipsychotics and antiemetics, has diverse properties resulting from the ability to block receptors for dopamine, histamine, noradrenaline, and acetylcholine to varying extents. It is not possible to generalize about their ability to provide or potentiate analgesia. Chlorpromazine is well described as being able to elevate pain threshold both in experimental animals and in man. It is less certain, however, that chlorpromazine produces useful analgesia in the clinical pain context or that it potentiates morphine analgesia (Houde 1966). Methotrimeprazine is an interesting anomaly in this class of drug in that it is capable of producing analgesia lasting approximately three hours in man, with 20 mg being approximately equivalent to 10 mg of morphine (both being given intramuscularly). In common with other phenothiazines it is sedative and can make patients very drowsy. It has been reported to cause severe orthostatic hypotension (Beaver *et al.* 1966). Other common side-effects of phenothiazines include blurred vision, dry mouth, tachycardia, and urinary retention.

The chief use of phenothiazines in the control of postoperative pain is likely to remain the relief of opioid-induced nausea and vomiting.

Butyrophenones are potent dopamine antagonist drugs with similar properties to the phenothiazines but have chemical resemblance to pethidine. Haloperidol is the best-known antipsychotic in the group, but droperidol is most commonly used intraoperatively in combination with fentanyl. Opinions vary as to the analgesic efficacy of these compounds (e.g. 'did not increase the analgesia produced by morphine but did reduce emesis' [Judkins & Harmer 1982] compared with 'will not only potentiate opiate analgesics but also show intrinsic analgesia' [Budd 1981]). Side-effects are broadly similar to the phenothiazines, but extrapyramidal effects are more likely and hallucinations have been recorded following high doses.

Benzodiazepines

This class of drug is able to relieve anxiety and produce sedation by modulating the affinity of the $GABA_A$ receptor for the inhibitory neurotransmitter gamma-aminobutyric acid (GABA). This results in potentiation of the action of this natural inhibitory substance. The relief of anxiety can be helpful to a patient in pain, but sedation can be troublesome. It is important to remember that some patients will become depressed following treatment with drugs of this type, and that the sedative effects of these agents are more pronounced when an opioid has been administered.

It is not clear whether diazepam and other benzodiazepines are capable of producing analgesia in the absence of other drugs but there is good evidence from animal studies that GABA-mimetic substances such as muscimol can produce spinal analgesia (Roberts *et al.* 1986).

Transmitter precursors and enzyme inhibitors

It has been known for some time that 5-hydroxytryptamine plays an important role in controlling the excitability of sensory neurones within the dorsal horn of the spinal cord. This descending pathway can be activated by systemic administration of opioids (*see* Chapter 5). The precursor of 5-hydroxytryptamine is an amino acid, 5-hydroxytryptophan, and administration of this substance will potentiate or prolong morphine analgesia. In one study, patients that had become tolerant to morphine again experienced good analgesia following 5-hydroxytryptophan. This type of therapy has limited application. An alternative strategy is to administer a substance that will prevent breakdown of transmitter substances. This will also work for peptides (where it is not possible to administer a precursor as they are not synthesized *de novo* but are cleaved from a polypeptide chain during post-translational processing). The principal target of research to date has been the enkephalin family, as they have a short biological half-life. The problem is not a simple one as there is no specific 'enkephalinase'. Three types of enzyme are involved in the metabolism of enkephalins — aminopeptidase, dipeptidylaminopeptidase, and a neutral endopeptidase. In animal experiments these can all be inhibited, and thus enkephalin can be potentiated to produce analgesia by giving a mixture of three or four enzyme inhibitors. This would obviously not be acceptable in the clinical context. Recently Roques and his colleagues (Fournie-Zaluski *et al.* 1984) have developed kelatorphan, a single drug that will act to inhibit the enzymes breaking down enkephalins. Kelatorphan produces analgesia in laboratory animals but is probably not sufficiently bioavailable to be a candidate for clinical use. A prodrug, acetorphan, has been made that is sufficiently well absorbed following systemic administration to inhibit brain enkephalin metabolism (Lecomte *et al.* 1986). This approach may lead to clinically useful analgesics.

Other agents

Painful skeletal muscle spasm can sometimes be relieved with dantrolene, which acts directly on the muscle fibres, probably by inhibition of calcium release from the sarcoplasmic reticulum within the cell. Baclofen, an agonist at the $GABA_B$ receptor, can also help muscle spasm. It acts within the spinal cord to reduce primary afferent transmitter release, and also has weak analgesic properties.

CHAPTER 8
The Pharmacology of Local Anaesthetics

The use of surgical local anaesthesia dates from the pioneering work on cocaine carried out in Vienna in the middle of the 19th century. In 1885, in the U.S.A., Corning described experiments in the dog in which epidural injection of cocaine produced loss of sensation below the segment of injection. This was followed by a similar administration to a human subject, which again resulted in profound analgesia below the site of injection. The use of cocaine for local anaesthesia has now virtually ceased, but the principles underlying current use of local anaesthetic drugs are broadly the same as those developed 100 years ago.

Site and mechanism of action

Drugs that are used as local anaesthetics will stabilize the excitable membranes of both nerve and muscle. When applied directly to a nerve local anaesthetics increase the threshold for action potential generation, slow the rate of rise of the action potential, and decrease the conduction velocity. Sufficiently high concentrations of drug will completely block transmission. Local anaesthetic drugs have little or no action on resting membrane potential. Detailed electrophysiological studies have shown that their action is due to blockade of the channels in the nerve membrane through which sodium ions flow to generate the fast inward current that produces the rising phase of the action potential.

Most clinically useful local anaesthetic drugs are either secondary or tertiary amines. At normal tissue pH between 5 and 20% of the drug is likely to be in its unionized form. This unionized drug is important, for it is only in this form that it can diffuse through the perineurium and other connective tissue in order to reach its site of action on the neuronal membrane. However, it is the charged form of the drug that is responsible for blocking the sodium channels.

The nature of the nerve fibre (whether motor or sensory)

seems to have little influence on the probability of blockade of transmission with a local anaesthetic. In practice, the smaller fibres tend to become blocked first, because they have a lesser capacity to maintain activity in the face of partial blockade, and because the drug diffuses through to them more easily. Most local anaesthetics show frequency dependence and will block an active nerve fibre more readily than an inactive one. This is because the local anaesthetic only gains access to the sodium channel when it is in its open state. This is in contrast to the action of the neurotoxin, tetrodotoxin, which will block the sodium channel in either its open or closed state.

Mechanism of unwanted actions

The most serious side-effect of local anaesthetics is cerebral excitation leading to convulsions. These agents will readily penetrate the blood−brain barrier should they gain access to the systemic circulation. They will then act on neurones within the brain in a manner similar to their action on peripheral neurones. Excitation and convulsions occur because the inhibitory interneurones are the first to be inactivated by the local anaesthetics (probably because they are tonically active and therefore have many of their sodium channels in the open state). The removal of inhibition leads to uncontrolled discharge of excitatory neurones. If sufficient drug has penetrated the brain then eventually all neuronal activity will cease. It should be remembered that cocaine is a special case and has an additional central stimulant action because it blocks the uptake of noradrenaline (*see* Chapter 7).

As mentioned earlier, muscle membrane can be depressed by local anaesthetics, and a number of drugs of this type are used as antidysrhythmics because of their ability to stabilize hyperexcitable cardiac tissue. In overdose local anaesthetics will produce myocardial depression. Smooth muscle is also depressed, and thus local anaesthetics are vasodilators. Cardiovascular collapse following overdose with these drugs is thus due to a mixture of cardiac and vascular effects.

Some individuals are hypersensitive to local anaesthetics and may therefore collapse due to anaphylaxis rather than by the mechanisms described above.

Methods for prolongation of action

It has been common practice to include a vasoconstrictor in solutions of local anaesthetic for many years. This is usually either adrenaline or noradrenaline in a concentration of 1 part in 100 000 or 200 000. The benefit of the vasoconstrictor is that it produces an increase in the time for which the local anaesthetic is in contact with the nerve before being carried away in the circulation. It is also possible that the use of vasoconstrictors reduces the effective systemic toxicity of local anaesthetics by controlling the rate at which the drug reaches the liver, thereby not overloading metabolic enzymes. There is a risk of producing cardiac dysrhythmias if solutions containing catecholamines are injected systemically. Synthetic analogues of vasopressin such as felypressin are sometimes used as alternative vasoconstrictors for this reason, as they do not have any action on the myocardium.

Practical aspects of when to use and when not to use vasoconstrictors are dealt with in a later chapter.

Individual agents

Cocaine

Although use is limited because of abuse liability and toxicity, cocaine solutions are still occasionally used topically for ophthalmic anaesthesia/analgesia. Cocaine paste is used for nasal perioperative analgesia, e.g. for polypectomy, and it can be used to produce blockade of the sphenopalatine ganglion across the mucosa of the side wall. The ability of cocaine to block noradrenaline uptake gives it intrinsic vasoconstrictor activity.

Lignocaine

This is the most commonly used local anaesthetic. It is more potent and longer lasting than procaine. In the absence of vasoconstrictors it is rapidly absorbed from the site of injection. Dizziness and drowsiness (possibly due to an active metabolite) are seen as side-effects.

Bupivacaine

This is a very potent local anaesthetic with a prolonged duration of action. It is otherwise similar to lignocaine, although considerably more toxic to the myocardium. Bupivacaine is some 10 times more potent than lignocaine at inhibiting the fast inward sodium current in rabbit isolated cardiac muscle fibres, and this effect lasts six times as long as that of lignocaine (Moller & Covino 1985). The clinical use of this drug in regional intravenous techniques has declined because of its cardiotoxicity. However, because bupivacaine is absorbed slowly into the systemic circulation from other sites of injection, its toxicity after, say, epidural or neurovascular sheath injection is no greater that that of other agents. The safety of drugs of this type depends on the relationship between the toxic concentration and the maximum concentration achieved after injection of the same volume of equi-effective concentrations of each drug.

Etidocaine

This is another long-acting local anaesthetic. It has been reported to be highly plasma protein-bound such that it will have little tendency to cross the placenta. In comparison with bupivacaine it is little used.

Prilocaine

This agent is of similar potency to lignocaine but has a shorter duration of action. High doses have a tendency to produce methaemoglobinaemia. It is used in accident and emergency situations because of its low acute toxicity.

Chloroprocaine

Chloroprocaine is similar to procaine and has found a use in obstetric practice because it is rapidly metabolized by plasma esterase and thus has little effect on the fetus. It has been reported to have a high neurotoxicity and its continued use is therefore open to question.

New developments

It would obviously be advantageous to develop a locally acting analgesic substance that selectively blocked transmission of information in nociceptive fibres without blocking large sensory afferents, or motor or autonomic fibres. The solution to this problem may come from research into the actions of a substance called capsaicin. This is the pungent, hot-tasting active ingredient of red peppers. The chemical structure is shown in Fig. 8.1. When capsaicin is injected into newborn rat pups it induces a selective and almost permanent degeneration of peptide-containing small sensory nerves, including those involved in pain transmission and in the mediation of the neurogenic inflammatory response. Capsaicin can also be applied topically to peripheral nerves of adult rats, and a similar long-lasting, apparently permanent, loss of sensory function results. Such perineural capsaicin treatment is advantageous, since it produces selective impairment of afferent nerve function supplying a particular organ or part of it. The clinical usefulness of capsaicin is, however, limited at present, since it is known from electrophysiological and animal studies to stimulate neuronal activity and will actually produce pain when first given. This excitation of the nerve endings is then followed by blocking of the sensory nerve, after which there is long-term selective neurotoxic impairment and irreversible cell destruction (Buck & Burks 1986). A number of capsaicin analogues have recently been developed and tested for analgesic/anti-inflammatory action. NE-19550 (Proctor & Gamble) is such an analogue (Fig. 8.1) and possesses oral and subcutaneous activity in animal analgesic tests and is claimed to have similar efficacy but a longer duration of action than morphine. Opioid, adrenergic, serotoninergic, dopaminergic, cholinergic, and GABAergic antagonists do not appear to affect NE-19550 analgesia, which also does not seem to be associated with the acute toxic or irreversible effects of capsaicin. NE-19550 has also been shown to inhibit prostaglandin synthesis, and this compound may represent a new class of non-narcotic analgesic.

The integrity of nerve endings both in the periphery and within the spinal cord relies on the transport of materials up and down the nerve, and it has been postulated that the use of axonal transport blockers (which disorganize microtubules within the

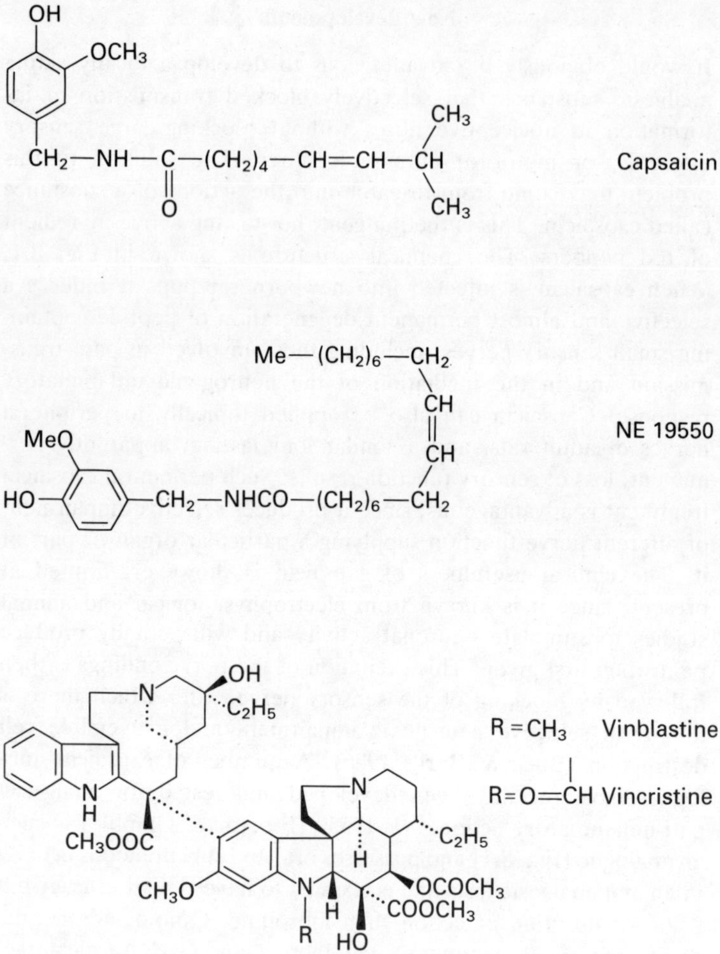

Capsaicin

NE 19550

R = CH$_3$ Vinblastine
R = O=CH   Vincristine

Fig. 8.1.

nerve) may be a new method to alleviate pain. Local application of these blockers (e.g. the antineoplastic vinca alkaloids, vincristine and vinblastine, [Fig. 8.1]) appears to be effective against a range of clinical intractable pain states, but pain relief is not total and problems in the administration of these drugs have been encountered.

CHAPTER 9

Choices in the Management of Postoperative Pain

Several decisions regarding the management of pain must be made. It is usual to use analgesic drugs to reduce, eliminate, or prevent pain. Can the use of these drugs be reduced by psychological preparation, by explanation and reassurance, or by additional care in the operation or in the perioperative period? Can they be reduced or replaced by transcutaneous nerve stimulation or by acupuncture or cryothermy? Should local anaesthetics or anti-inflammatory analgesics be used to reduce the perception of the noxious stimuli, or should narcotic analgesics be used systemically or regionally to reduce the feeling of pain? When should analgesics be given — when the patient asks for pain relief, or before the pain becomes apparent? Who is the best person to administer pain relief — the nurse, who is present all the time, the resident doctor or the pain specialist, who is able to relieve pain in a greater number of ways, or the patient, who is the one who knows how severe the pain is? These and other questions can only be answered by consideration of:
1 The availability of drugs, equipment, expertise, and time of the medical and nursing staff.
2 The disability, disease, concomitant drugs, and rate of deterioration of the patient.
3 The severity, character, and site of the pain.

Supervision of analgesia

The availability of methods of analgesia depends upon the level of patient care and monitoring. Effective analgesia depends upon being able to give sufficient drug to relieve the pain, but not enough to cause complications. Since patients vary in the amounts required, the inadequacy or overdosage of pain relief is determined by assessing the patients at intervals following the administration of the drug. If the pain can be controlled by small doses of paracetamol or the non-steroidal anti-inflammatory drugs given at infrequent intervals, the level of monitoring required is low. If the pain is sufficient to warrant continuous administration of narcotic analgesics or the use of epidural anaesthesia, the level required is much higher.

If the level of staffing is such that the patients' pain cannot be treated immediately, giving analgesia when the need arises (*pro re nata,* p.r.n.) is a very inefficient method. Either the drug will be given in high dosage to prolong its effect, and therefore cause relative overdosage at the time of its peak effect, or there will be periods of increasing pain before each administration. The 'p.r.n.' or 'on-demand' prescription is especially difficult to administer, since demands by each patient occur, and must be responded to, at irregular intervals. The demand itself represents inadequate analgesia, the cumulative effect of preceding doses is difficult to assess, and the administration of drugs, especially controlled drugs, is time-consuming and usually delayed. It is actually less time-consuming to offer analgesics to all postoperative patients at relatively frequent intervals.

The greater the effect of the analgesic technique, the greater the need for monitoring, but bolus injections of powerful drugs with either a rapid action or a delayed onset present the greatest need for intensive monitoring. The resistance to, or decline of, postoperative epidural local anaesthesia is due mainly to the rapidity with which postural hypotension may occur, and the technique is now almost confined to the intensive therapy, recovery, and delivery units. Other local anaesthetic techniques, such as intercostal blockade, are associated with complications, e.g. pneumothorax, which may become apparent minutes or hours after the blockade, and these too require prolonged monitoring.

If the staff involved in the active administration of analgesics have a thorough understanding of the drugs and methods of administration, the efficacy of the analgesics can be improved without further risk. The diagnosis of the pain and its cause, the use of the appropriate analgesic, the adjustment of the dose regimen of the drug to fit the response of the patient, the knowledge of interactions between agonists and partial agonists or between analgesics and concomitant drugs, and the methods of slow or controlled administration, all improve the safety of pain management. Medical staff could be more involved in the management of pain, not only in the prescription of drugs, but in the monitoring of response and frequent adjustment of dose, timing, or rate of administration to match the varying levels of pain, and in the use of local anaesthetic techniques.

The patient, too, can be instrumental in the relief of his pain, not only by avoiding reticence or exaggeration in describing the pain, but also by the self-administration of analgesics. The patient-controlled inhalational and intravenous analgesic devices have not proved to be more unsafe or more liable to abuse than most other methods of analgesia.

The availability of the methods of analgesia dependent upon the availability of personnel is shown in Table 9.1.

However, it is probable that pain is managed more efficiently in recovery rooms, specialized postoperative wards, and intensive therapy units, not only because of increased staff–patient ratios and increased staff expertise, but also because the problem of postoperative pain is considered more frequently, and more effort and ingenuity are used to combat it.

Disability, disease, and drugs of the patient

The diseases and conditions which influence the choice of drug or dosage are considered in Table 9.2. Most of the drugs which interact with the analgesic drugs are tabulated in Appendix I.

Character, site, and severity of the pain

The factors which influence the severity of postoperative pain are considered in Chapter 3. Pain arises within stimulated, inflamed, damaged, or ischaemic somatic tissues, by traction of mesenteries and fasciae, and from the distension of hollow viscera. Some organs, such as the lung and liver, appear to be unable to cause pain when stimulated.

Most inflammatory or traumatic pains are made worse by movement and can be improved by immobilization and by reducing the tissue pressure by, say, elevation of the part. However, whereas the limbs may be immobilized, the trunk cannot be without impairing the ventilation. Visceral distension or spasm is frequently accompanied by somatic muscle spasm ('guarding'), and both can be very painful. Postoperative pain is usually most severe when it involves the abdomen and thorax, especially in

Table 9.1. Administrators of postoperative analgesia.

Personnel	Advantages	Disadvantages	Methods available
Nurse	Almost immediately available on the ward Continuous monitoring of patient demand/behaviour may be possible	Not trained to diagnose all types of pain Methods of analgesia very limited	Reassurance, physical methods of pain relief, e.g. massage, adjustment of dressing Demonstration of care
Trained nurse	Continuous monitoring may be possible	Not always immediately available, especially at night Not trained to diagnose all types of pain Cannot change prescription	As above plus oral, intramuscular, subcutaneous, and rectal administration of drugs regularly or on demand
Generalist doctor	Often available on ward except at night Always available for discussion or diagnosis Knows preoperative state, diagnosis, and prognosis Trained to diagnose extraoperative pain Can titrate analgesia against pain Can alter the prescription	Trained in fewer methods of pain relief than specialist Less available than nurse May be engaged in theatre for several hours	As above plus intravenous bolus or infusion, local infiltration, 'top-up' of continuous local anaesthesia, or spinal opioid analgesia

specialist doctor in anaesthesia or pain relief	Knows diagnosis and prognosis Trained to recognize and diagnose extraoperative pain Can titrate analgesia against pain Trained in most forms of pain management Wide knowledge of pharmacokinetics and pharmacodynamics of analgesics Able to change prescription	Not always available at short notice except in intensive therapy units and recovery rooms Not available to monitor patient continuously Reliant on reports of pain state and response	As above plus institution of all forms of local anaesthesia and spinal opioid analgesia Transcutaneous nerve stimulation Sometimes accupuncture and hypnosis Dissociative analgesia e.g. ketamine Continuous inhalational analgesia Profound analgesia with ventilatory or haemodynamic support
Patient	Always available Intimate knowledge of site, character, severity, and onset of pain	May not know diagnosis/prognosis Cannot change prescription Poor knowledge (usually) of latency of onset of analgesic — may become impatient for result Administration of analgesic depends on the awake state	Oral drugs as prescribed when out-patient Patient-controlled inhalational analgesia, e.g. Entonox Patient-controlled intravenous analgesic via, for example, Cardiff Palliator

Table 9.2. Conditions of the patient that affect the choice of analgesic or techniques.

Condition	Analgesic affected	Effect
Liver disease		
Hypoproteinaemia	Paracetamol	Dose-dependent toxicity.
	All	Reduced plasma protein binding: effects increased
Reduced clotting factors	NSAIDs	All cause gastric irritation, and tendency to haematemesis is increased. Some, e.g. aspirin, reduce prothrombin levels more than others, e.g. naproxen
	Mefenamic acid Indomethacin	May cause thrombocytopenia
	Local anaesthetic	Invasive techniques more likely to cause haemorrhage. Intraspinal haemorrhage may cause paraplegia. Techniques in which bleeding cannot be controlled should not be used
Fluid overload, e.g. oedema, ascites	Indomethacin Piroxicam Phenylbutazone	Increase fluid retention
Hepatic encephalopathy	Opioids	Increased narcosis; constipation increases absorption of toxins
	Mefenamic acid	May cause haemolysis and cholestatic jaundice
Renal disease	All	Excretion delayed

Table 9.2. *Continued.*

Condition	Analgesic affected	Effect
Renal disease *continued*	Pethidine	Increase of norpethidine may cause tachycardia, convulsions
	Morphine Diamorphine Papaveretum	Morphine 6-glucuronide accumulates; this is potent and causes prolonged narcotic analgesia and ventilatory depression
	NSAIDs Paracetamol	Increased fluid retention and deterioration of renal function
	Aspirin Diflunisal	Cumulation, therefore increased risk of gastrointestinal bleeding
Addiction	Opioids	Tolerance developed, larger doses required
Asthma	NSAIDs	Hypersensitivity may present as bronchospasm
	Opioids	Release histamine — may provoke bronchospasm
	Local anaesthetics	Usually help to relieve bronchospasm via systemic effect
Anxiety/fear	Local anaesthetics plus adrenaline	Tachycardia potential
	Aspirin	Increased metabolic rate: additive effects
	Ketamine Nefopam	Increased release of sympathetic amines: synergism

Table 9.2. Continued.

Condition	Analgesic affected	Effect
Anxiety/fear *continued*	Opioids	More drug required for same effect
	Local anaesthesia	Touch, pressure may be interpreted as pain
	All	Pain threshold reduced
Addison disease	Opioids Spinal anaesthesia	Hypotension and hypotensive crises may be precipitated
Age — *see* Appendix III		
Breast feeding — *see also* Appendix III	Morphine	More potent in neonate or premature infant because of immature blood–brain barrier but single therapeutic maternal doses unlikely to affect infant adversely
Colic, renal, biliary	Opioids	May increase smooth muscle spasm — effect reduced by hyoscine, xanthines, and glyceryl trinitrate
Diabetes mellitus (monitoring of)	Opioids	Blood sugar raised
	Paracetamol	Blood sugar lowered
	Indomethacin Large doses of salicylates	Blood sugar raised, glycosuria. NB postoperative stress also changes blood glucose levels
Epilepsy	Pethidine Nefopam	Increased likelihood of convulsions

Table 9.2. *Continued.*

Condition	Analgesic affected	Effect
Glaucoma	Ketamine Nefopam	Increase intraocular pressure
Gout	Aspirin	Low doses cause retention of uric acid, high doses are uricosuric; inhibits action of probenecid
Head injury	Opioids	Depress ventilation: high doses increase carbon dioxide levels and indirectly increase cerebral blood flow and intracranial pressure. Monitoring of level of consciousness and pupil size more difficult
	Ketamine	Raises intracranial pressure
	Nefopam	May cause hypertension and raise intracranial pressure
Hypertension	Ketamine	Increases blood pressure
	Nefopam	May increase blood pressure
	Opioids	High doses may cause sudden hypotension in untreated patients, especially those who are renin-resistant
Hyperthyroidism	Aspirin, etc.	Increase metabolic rate. Compete with thyroxine for protein-binding sites: potentiation
	Fenclofenac Phenylbutazone	Give a false low total plasma thyroxine concentration
	Opioids	More drug required for same effect

Table 9.2. *Continued.*

Condition	Analgesic affected	Effect
Hyperthyroidism *continued*	Adrenaline in local anaesthetics	Potentiation — may lead to hyperthyroid crisis, ventricular fibrillation
Hypothyroidism	All	Reduced metabolism — increased effect. Slow circulation time — increased effect of bolus doses
Hypovolaemia/shock	All	Regional blood flow altered: absorption delayed; systemic drugs should be given intravenously
	Opioids	Hypotensive effect potentiated. Naloxone may cause clinical improvement
	Local anaesthetics	Heart rate slowed, vasoconstriction reversed depending on dose used. Sympathetic blockade, e.g. spinal techniques, potentiates hypotension
Hypothermia	Epidural, intrathecal anaesthetic	Causes widespread vasodilation and heat loss. Shivering reduced by concurrent narcosis
Infection	Local anaesthetics	May spread infection — including fungal infection. Less effective and more toxic in inflamed tissues
	Opioids	May increase septic shock syndrome. Naloxone should be considered for treatment

Table 9.2. *Continued.*

Condition	Analgesic affected	Effect
Lung disease including obesity, chronic obstructive airway disease, and fibrosis	Opioids	Reduced respiratory reserve. hypercarbia reduces sensitivity of respiratory centre — ventilatory depression more likely
	Local anaesthesia: spinal, intercostal	Reduces power of inspiratory intercostal muscles and reduces respiratory capacity further. NB Pain also respiratory depressant
Morbid obesity	Opioids	Altered level of endogenous opioids — increased tendency to narcosis and reduced sensitivity to airway occlusion potentiated by exogenous opioids
Myocardial infarction	Pentazocine Butorphanol	Cardiac work increased — extension of infarction possible
	Ketamine	Contractility depressed but noradrenaline levels increased
	Adrenaline, etc.	Increase myocardial excitability, arrhythmias more likely
Myotonia, myasthenia, etc.	Opioids	Decreased respiratory power — potentiation of ventilatory depression
Multiple sclerosis	Opioids	Greater risk from ventilatory depression
Peptic ulceration	NSAIDs	Increased risk of bleeding even when given systemically

Table 9.2. *Continued.*

Condition	Analgesic affected	Effect
Plasma cholinesterase deficiency	Ester-type local anaesthetics	Prolongation of action
Pregnancy	Aspirin and other NSAIDs	Impaired platelet function. Increased haemorrhage. Kernicterus in jaundiced neonates. High doses may close the ductus arteriosus *in utero* leading to pulmonary hypertension in the newborn. Delay in onset and duration of labour, haemorrhage more likely
	Opioids	Depress neonatal respiration, cause gastric stasis and nausea — increased risk of inhalation pneumonitis during labour
	Morphine	Prolongs labour. Antioxytocic
	Pethidine Pentazocine	Increases effect of oxytocics. No effect on activity of normally contracting uterus.
	Methadone	No effect on uterus at term
	Morphine Methadone	Equianalgesic doses are more depressant to the neonate than pethidine, fentanyl, etc.
Prostatic hypertrophy	Opioids, especially morphine	Central and peripheral effect causing urinary retention
	Spinal anaesthetic	Urinary retention
Sleep apnoea, snoring	Opioids	Respiratory arrest more likely

Table 9.2. *Continued.*

Condition	Analgesic affected	Effect
Smoking	Opioids	Tolerance to opioids
Terminal care	Opioids	Dependence is not a consideration. Complications such as ventilatory depression must be weighed against a shortened life expectation

association with convulsive movements such as sneezing or coughing. Such pain is not readily relieved by systemic analgesics and can be abolished only by local anaesthesia.

Pain arising from compressed or damaged nerves may require more than NSAIDs for relief. Any very severe pain, pain exaggerated by anxiety, and pain which has persisted for a long time requires narcotic analgesics, local anaesthesia, or some other method of altering the interpretation of pain mentioned above. Pain which results from damage of the neural pathways may be treated more effectively not by conventional analgesics, but by drugs which affect the central modulating pathways, such as the anticonvulsants, the tricyclic antidepressants, or the sedatives.

Conversely, NSAIDs may be capable of eliminating pains such as dental pain, dysmenorrhoea, and some bone pain, whereas the narcotic analgesics only reduce their severity. Indeed, the pain following removal of the wisdom teeth, especially when coronitis is already present, has been shown to be relieved more effectively by aspirin than by dihydrocodeine.

Sharp pain or crescendo pain, such as is present during labour, can be relieved rather than reduced by local anaesthesia, and by opioids, but only by the very high concentrations of opioids achieved by intrathecal administration.

Visceral muscle spasm, e.g. urinary catheter spasm or biliary duct spasm, may also be difficult to relieve by conventional analgesics but responds well to antispasmodics such as atropine, hyoscine, or glyceryl trinitrate.

Pain from phantom limbs is not relieved by local anaesthesia of the part. It may even be increased. However, a more proximal nerve block, which involves the appropriate sympathetic supply, may be successful, as may the use of narcotic analgesics, transcutaneous electrical nerve stimulation, or the neuromodulating drugs mentioned above.

The *site* of pain determines also the feasibility of local anaesthesia. Cannulation of the space around cranial nerves is difficult, that of the cervical epidural space carries considerable risk. Local anaesthetic techniques may be contraindicated because of infection or soiling and be technically difficult if the painful part lies beneath thick bandages, or is very extensive or geographically diverse. For example, the discomfort arising from a nasogastric tube, an intravenous infusion in the upper limb, and an abdominoperineal wound is difficult to relieve with subtoxic doses of local anaesthetic.

The site, severity, and character of the pain may be used to diagnose the cause of pain in the postoperative period, for it must not be assumed that all postoperative pain arises from the damaged tissues. Some may be due to ischaemic tissues because of constrictive dressings or emboli, to a full bladder, or because of nerve entrapment. The advent of a new pain is a cause of concern, it may be a warning of further damage and, in general, postoperative pain should be treated when the cause is established.

The *time-course* and *strength* of the analgesia should match that of the pain. Some pains are continuous, e.g. abdominal pain, injuries to ligaments, pressure within an organ such as bladder distension, or glaucoma. Other pains are intermittent or do not occur in every case. Inguinal herniorrhaphy is followed by moderate to severe pain in only 30–70% of patients, depending upon the surgical and anaesthetic techniques and the country of reporting. Some pains of muscle spasm can be relieved as effectively by a centrally acting muscle relaxant as by an opioid, although care should be exercised when using both drugs together, since the sedative and ventilatory depressant effects may be increased.

Methods of analgesia

The effects of the timing of the method of analgesia are compared in Table 9.3.

Table 9.3. The timing of analgesia.

	Advantages	Disadvantages
Intermittent on demand	Provided frequency limited, method unlikely to cause overdosage Method suitable for pain of irregular severity Flexible, therefore simple to prescribe, requiring little, if any, adjustment Analgesia is managed by the nursing staff Minimal equipment required	Pain demand occurs when pain intolerable: response to demand rarely immediate and effective analgesia delayed Patient in pain for considerable periods As each demand of each patient occurs irregularly, wasteful of nurses' time
Regular	Analgesia independent of patient's stoicism and nursing response to analgesic demand Simple and convenient to administer and is more economical of nurses' time Reduced patient anxiety of persistent or prolonged pain Usually gives more effective relief than demand analgesia	Analgesics given in absence of pain so that accumulation, overdosage and emergence of side-effects possible Monitoring required The greater the interval of administration, the wider the swing from pain to relative overdosage Pain diminishes with time and prescription must be adjusted May mask pain arising from other causes
Continuous	Analgesia continuous and not subject to the fluctuations of the above methods. It is possible to maintain the analgesic corridor between pain and unpleasant, unwanted side-effects	Does not cope with changing severity of pain or changing tolerance May mask pain arising from other causes Requires monitoring and adjustments to achieve and maintain adequate analgesic, non-toxic levels

Table 9.3. *Continued*

	Advantages	Disadvantages
Continuous *continued*		Requires apparatus which restricts patient movement and which may be a source of infection
Patient-controlled analgesia	Immediate response to pain possible, thereby altering the analgesia to suit the pain Suitable for pain of varying intensity; reduces patient anxiety with regard to pain Overdosage and persistence of unpleasant side-effects unlikely	Patient responds only to pain which is already present, therefore pain not completely prevented Requires motivation and action by patient who may be restricted or apathetic Pain relief not available when asleep or confused Equipment costly
Pre-emptive offer or administration, i.e. the nurse offers analgesics prior to painful procedures or regularly at short intervals	Timing of drugs convenient Pain tolerance not reached and concern demonstrated Minimal equipment required Assessment before each dose — overdosage unlikely	Few disadvantages, but depends on nursing staff being available and making assessments before demands made Analgesia not continuous and dose may have to be adjusted

Choice of analgesic drug and technique

Although surgically induced pain *can* be reduced by non-drug methods, drugs are almost invariably used to relieve pain in the postoperative period. Opioids are most frequently used for visceral or severe pain, and non-steroidal anti-inflammatory agents or paracetamol for pain of inflammatory origin. Local anaesthesia

Choices in Management of Postoperative Pain

is used in suitable cases where sufficient expertise and monitoring exist, and inhalational agents are sometimes used for short-term pain or painful procedures. Other potent analgesics exist, such as ketamine, which can relieve severe pain, and it is frequently true that a combination of drugs or methods of analgesia can relieve pain more effectively or with less risk than any one drug or method used in isolation.

The relative advantages of local and general analgesia are noted in Table 9.4. The choice of local anaesthetic and local anaesthetic technique is discussed in the next chapter. It should be noted that the advantages of both methods can be combined when the somatic, or dermatomusculoskeletal, element of the pain is relieved by a local anaesthetic technique and the visceral element by the general analgesics applied systemically, or even regionally.

The advantages and disadvantages of the use of spinal opioids are discussed in the Chapter 11.

The routes of administration of the systemic analgesics are compared in Table 9.5.

Notes on methods of systemic analgesia

Oral administration

This is a convenient form of administration. The drug is not

Table 9.4. A comparison of local anaesthesia and systemic analgesia.

	Local anaesthesia	Systemic analgesia
Pain at the operative site	Can relieve all kinds of pain: sharp and dull, constant and convulsive; prevents muscle spasm	Opioids can relieve all kinds of pain only at very high dosage and with medullary depression. Therapeutic doses relieve dull pain much more than sharp pain or pain occasioned by movement. NSAIDs relieve sharp and dull pain but not that of great severity

Table 9.4. *Continued.*

	Local anaesthesia	Systemic analgesia
Generalized discomfort	Does not relieve pain outside the area of nerve blockade	Relieves discomfort from other causes, e.g. intravenous drip site, nasogastric tube, pressure sores
Anxiety	Does not allay anxiety except by relief of pain	Allays anxiety (opioids)
Administration	The initial administration is invasive, and demands considerable skill and sterile conditions, which are not always readily available. The invasive administration may be painful or technically difficult because of the site of the operative wound. Cannulation reduces many of the difficulties of repeated administration	Less skill required: can be administered by nurses, therefore more readily available Administration causes little if any pain
Side-effects	Local complications such as infection, bruising, nerve damage Systemic complications such as sympathetic blockade, causing hypotension, bradycardia, loss of heat, cardiac arrhythmias, loss of function of limbs or bladder, tolerance and tachyphylaxis	Opioids: ventilatory depression, nausea and vomiting, itching, ileus, retention of urine, tolerance NSAIDs: increased bleeding, gastric irritation, retention of fluid Paracetamol: impaired liver function
Principal advantages	Superior pain relief Allows effective coughing in the presence of abdominal or thoracic wound pain No diminution of consciousness	Ease of administration More readily available

Choices in Management of Postoperative Pain 119

Route of administration	Proportion of drug absorbed into systemic circulation	Rate of absorption[1]	Effect of stress, anxiety, shock or hypotension	Is sterility required?	Advantages
Intravenous	All — directly	Immediate	Higher proportion of drug delivered to heart and brain — reduced rate of metabolism and excretion	Yes	Most rapid and reliable form of administration. Does can be titrated against pain. It is the preferred route in shock, as absorption does not depend on regional blood flow. Rapid effect makes it suitable for patient-controlled analgesia (PCA)
Intramuscular	All — directly	Moderate	Absorption delayed	Yes	Absorption slower, peak effect less, and duration of effect longer
Subcutaneous	All — directly	Slow — can be varied	Absorption greatly delayed	Yes	Effect even more constant and prolonged than above
Transdermal	Variable unless occlusive dressing used — directly	Slow	Absorption greatly delayed	No	Non-invasive, painless administration
Oral	Very variable — via portal circulation and liver	Moderate to slow — rate can be reduced by slow-release preparations	Absorption delayed to a variable extent[2]	No	Non-invasive, painless, easy to administer[3], relatively inexpensive, no additional equipment required
Sublingual	Variable depending on how much of the dose is swallowed — directly	Moderate	Absorption slightly delayed	No	Relatively inexpensive tablet form which enters the systemic circulation directly
Nasal	Slightly variable, some may be exhaled — directly	Moderate to rapid	Little effect	No	Convenient administration, which enters the systemic circulation directly
Pulmonary	Variable, most of the gas is expired, — directly	Rapid	Slight — because of altered ventilation–perfusion ratio	No	Rapid onset of peak effect, Self-administration device inherently safe because of the need to make an airtight seal to inhale gas at subatmospheric pressure
Rectal	Variable, some may be evacuated before absorption, — directly	Moderate	Delayed, but less than with oral route	No	Suitable for conscious or unconscious patient

Table 9.5. *Continued.*

Route of Administration	Disadvantages	Appropriate person to administer drug	Analgesic techniques feasible by this route	Drugs available by this route
Intravenous	Onset of peak rate of biotransformation and excretion also rapid, therefore duration of effect relatively short. Requires trained staff to administer drug, therefore drug may not be immediately available.	Doctor or patient (for PCA)	Bolus injection on demand Regular bolus injections Continuous on computer-controlled infusions Patient-controlled analgesia (PCA)	Opioids Some NSAIDs, e.g. lysine acid salicylate, ketorolac Nefopam, ketamine
Intramuscular	Rate of absorption dependent on regional blood flow to muscle; some drugs painful on injection, e.g. diclofenac. Pain more likely when muscles wasted. Risk of inadvertent vascular or neural puncture. Concurrent anticoagulation may lead to extensive bruising	Doctor or nurse	Bolus injection on demand Regular bolus injections	Opioids Some NSAIDs e.g. lysine acid salicylate, ketorolac, diclofenac Nefopam, ketamine
Subcutaneous	Rate of absorption dependent on skin blood flow and even more dependent than above on shock, anxiety, sedation, or hypoventilation. Some irritant drugs cause ulcers or abscesses	Doctor or nurse	Bolus injection on demand[a] Regular bolus injections Continuous infusions	Opioids ketamine
Transdermal	Absorption too slow to allow titration of drug against pain Few drugs available for this use	Doctor, nurse or patient	Regular application	Hyoscine (for muscle spasm) Glyceryl trinitrate (for angina), fentanyl
Oral	In the postoperative period, the patient may be stuporous or the laryngeal reflexes may be sluggish. Oral administration may then lead to inhalation of the drug. Oral ingestion may cause nausea and vomiting. Gastric emptying may be delayed following stress, pain, opioids, or anaesthesia: absorption from the small intestine would be delayed. Gastric irritants, e.g. aspirin, more irritant to the empty stomach	Doctor, nurse or patient	On demand or regular administration	Paracetamol NSAIDs Opioids Ketamine

Sublingual	Excessive salivation leads to swallowing. Like the oral route, this route is not safe unless the larynx is competent. Few drugs are available for this route of absorption	Doctor, nurse or patient	On demand or regular administration	Buprenorphine, phenazocine, glyceryl trinitrate
Nasal	Drugs must be in fine powder or mist form. Conscious effort required. Inappropriate during bouts of the common cold or if mucosa altered by cocaine	Patient	On demand or regular administration	Diamorphine, morphine and cocaine 'snorted' by addict population
Pulmonary	Bulky equipment required. Effect short-lasting. Dry gases lead to retrosternal soreness. Hyperventilation leads to dizziness. Exhaled gases cause environmental contamination. Continuous administration needs continuous supervision	Patient/nurse: physiotherapist for PCA: anaesthetist for continuous	On demand administration Continuous administration Patient-controlled analgesia	Nitrous oxide/oxygen Tricholoroethylene[5] morphine, diamorphine[6]
Rectal	Proportion of dose unknown, especially when intestinal hurry present. Application may initiate evacuation. May cause proctitis. Aesthetically unpleasing to the majority of British patients	Doctor, nurse, patient	On demand or regular administration	Some NSAIDs e.g. indomethacin, piroxicam Some opioids, e.g. morphine, dextromoramide

Choices in Management of Postoperative Pain   121

Notes

1 This depends not only on the route of administration but also on the solubility and dissociation constant of the drug, the acidity of the environment, and the surface area and the regional blood flow of the absorptive area.
2 Systemic absorption from the gastrointestinal tract depends on:
a The site of absorption — stomach or small intestine.
b The rate of passage and dissolution of the drug in a patient who may be dehydrated and recumbent.
c The rate of gastric emptying.
d The amount of drug which traverses the hepatic circulation without biotransformation.
3 Unless the patient is uncooperative, in which case great skill is required.
4 The insertion of a plastic, low-volume cannula subcutaneously in children during the operative procedure and general anaesthetic allows painless postoperative injection of many drugs.
5 Tricholoroethylene, although more long-lasting than nitrous oxide, is rarely used because of the induced nausea, tachycardia and tachypnoea.
6 In the 19th century, the distillation and inhalation of opium was used by postoperative patients (and their attendants), but now morphine and diamorphine are smoked only by the addict population (chasing the dragon).

required to be sterile. The nurse or the patient can administer the drug. It is the most convenient, and sometimes the only feasible, form of administration of analgesia following out-patient surgery.

Following general anaesthesia, ketamine anaesthesia, or oral surgery under local anaesthesia, the laryngeal reflexes may be incompetent for several hours, and part of the medication may be aspirated. In the recumbent position, insoluble tablets may lodge in the oesophagus and remain unabsorbed. If gastric stasis occurs as a result of the surgery, the stress, or because of administered opioids etc., the drug may not reach the principal absorptive site of the small intestine for many hours. Not only does this result in delayed analgesia, but it may be the cause of overdosage if delayed effective passage coincides in time with the administration of subsequent doses.

Intermittent, on demand, administration

Drugs can be administered by a number of routes (*see* Table 9.5) but the amount of drug absorbed through the skin, the lungs, or the mucosa of the buccal, nasal, or rectal cavity is uncertain. Injection into blood, muscle, or subcutaneous tissue is usually preferred.

Intermittent administration on demand depends on the patient's intolerance of the pain, the lack of confusion, the availability of attending staff, the legal procedures to be followed, and the further delay before the drug exerts its maximal effect. Because of these difficulties there is a tendency to prescribe larger than ideal doses so that the duration of effect is increased. The patient oscillates between pain and overdose. Conversely, the method is versatile. It is suitable to be prescribed for the patient who has irregular or occasional pain or who has no pain at all. Accumulation of drug is unlikely to occur.

Continuous administration

Continuous analgesia can be achieved by long-acting drugs such as piroxicam, but is usually maintained by repeated or continuous administration, such that the drug is given before the preceding dose has declined to subanalgesic levels. This technique is es-

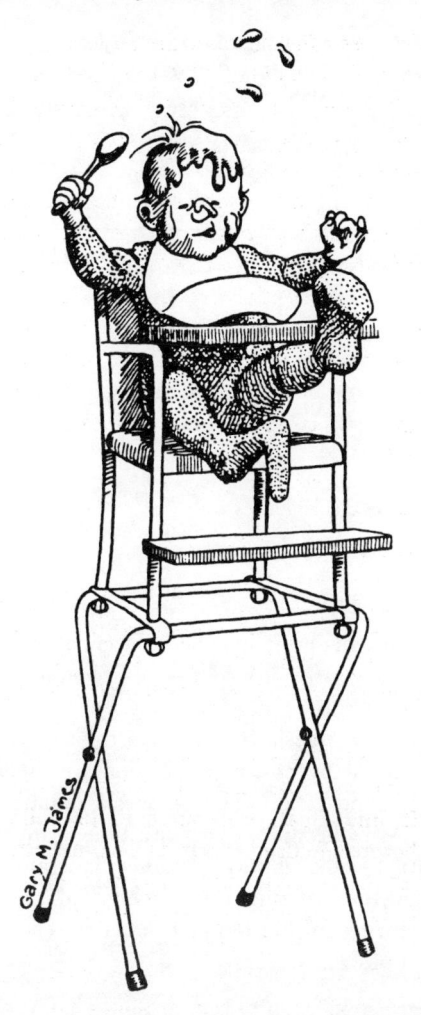

Oral administration is suitable only for the conscious and co-operative patient.

pecially valuable for short-acting drugs or where it is desirable to maintain the drug at low concentration (e.g. ketamine). The larger the dose and the faster the onset and offset of action, the greater the oscillations of analgesia. The smaller the dose and the greater the frequency of administration, the more completely will the effect travel the analgesic corridor (Fig. 9.1) between pain and

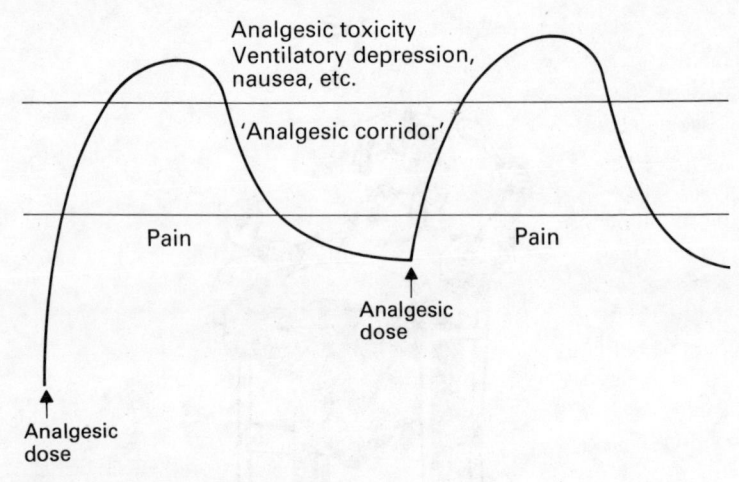

Fig. 9.1. The analgesic corridor.

toxic overdosage. The acme of systemic analgesia for continuous pain is continuous analgesia matched to the patients' requirement. This can be achieved by infusion — intravenous, subcutaneous, epidural, or intrathecal. Infusions may be preceded by loading doses, to achieve analgesia, from which the steady state is maintained, or followed by a second infusion which declines as the steady state is approached. The analgesic requirements of each patient varies with the operation, with time, with the pain tolerance, and with the distribution volumes and rate of elimination of the drug by the patient. The response of the patient needs constant monitoring so that the pain remains relieved and so that accumulation does not occur.

Patient-controlled analgesia

Since the patient knows how severe the pain is and when it occurs, it is logical to allow him to achieve and maintain analgesia.

Entonox demand analgesia

A 50% mixture of nitrous oxide in oxygen can provide effective analgesia in most patients in most circumstances. The patient demand apparatus delivers the gas only when an airtight fit is maintained between the face and the mask or mouthpiece. If the patient becomes somnolent or confused, the airtight fit will be lost and the gas flow will cease. Recovery from the effect of the gas is rapid. The technique is therefore inherently safe. An analgesic level is reached, in most cases, after four deep breaths, and can be maintained by intermittent inhalations from the device. However, since the effect is short-lived, it is tiring to use to maintain a constant level of analgesia. The gas is dry, and prolonged use can lead to retrosternal soreness. The apparatus is cumbersome, and patient mobility is limited. Effective analgesia depends upon the patient's understanding and co-ordination. Thus, although Entonox can be used alone to provide effective analgesia even after upper abdominal surgery, its availability is more valuable for short painful procedures such as dressing changes or physiotherapy. Although it has been shown that prolonged ventilation of nitrous oxide−oxygen mixtures is associated with falls of the white cell count, in practice the postoperative consumption of Entonox is very small. Trichloroethylene inhalers are now rarely used for postoperative pain.

Intravenous patient-controlled analgesia

A device for injecting a preset dose of analgesic into an intravenous infusion was developed by Sechzer (1968). A delay timer was incorporated so that each successful demand was followed by a refractory period in which no further drug could be delivered. This allowed each bolus of drug to achieve an effect before the delivery of subsequent doses and helped to prevent overdosage by impatience. Later devices incorporated controls of the background infusion and other fail-safe mechanisms.

The Cardiff Palliator is a simple robust device with some advantages. It incorporates a digitally driven syringe pump which adds drug to an infusion line. The dose is preset and, since the syringe must be refilled manually, the total amount available is also determined. The refractory period is variable to take account of the variable pharmacokinetics of different drugs, and there is an additional safety mechanism in the demand switch. This switch is a press button which must be depressed twice in one second to be effective; this eliminates most of the danger of accidental activation by body pressure, falls, etc. The doses are set in milligrams rather than drops.

A further advance was made in the design of the ODAC (on-demand analgesic computer) in that a background infusion of the drug can be maintained, the rate of which can be made dependent on the number of analgesic demands. As more demands are made, the rate of infusion increases, so that the effort of repeated demands for analgesia is diminished. Most of these machines are mains-driven, albeit with a battery back-up, but some newer smaller devices are becoming available which are more portable, allowing the patient more freedom of movement.

The patient-controlled analgesia (PCA) device may inject into an existing infusion, or directly into a vein. If an infusion is used, it is easier to determine when the cannula has become dislodged from the vein or has become blocked. The extravasation, unless large, is clinically unimportant since the drug will continue to be absorbed from the subcutaneous site; the delay in analgesic effect will prompt more analgesic demands. However, if the infusion becomes blocked the drug increments would accumulate in the blocked infusion to be administered together when the blockage is resolved. Modern devices with pressure limit warnings indicate blockage only when the block is in the device or its own delivery systems.

Almost all those reporting on the use of PCA devices show improvement compared to on-demand, nurse-administered analgesia. One study which failed to show an improvement (Ellis *et al.* 1982) also reported unusually low pain scores and a high frequency of nurse-administered analgesia in the control group.

The principal advantage is that, as the patient is controlling the analgesia, the pain should be reduced to tolerable levels. Respiratory depression does not appear to be a problem, except when buprenorphine is used (Gibbs *et al.* 1982), despite a wide range in the number of demands and total amount of drug delivered. The disadvantages are many. When the pain is spasmodic, the method is unlikely to be helpful and may lead to toxicity. Because the individual doses are small, analgesia may require many demands over a significant period. Since the demands are initiated by pain, some pain is likely to be present for most of the time. If the drug is rapid in its onset and offset, the frequency of demand is high (almost 12 per hour for alfentanil [Kay 1981]). During confusion or sleep demands will not be made despite the consequences of noxious stimuli in terms of vasoconstriction, truncated breathing, etc. Furthermore, some patients become lethargic or apathetic (acquired helplessness) and given a choice of movement and deep breathing made possible after a voluntary effort of demand analgesia or lying motionless to avoid pain will choose the latter. The ODAC and King's Pain Recorder communicate with the patient and demand a response.

Other forms of analgesia

Acupuncture

Despite many reports of the use of acupuncture for postoperative pain, it remains an unusual form of postoperative analgesia in the West, and controlled clinical trials are few. Sung *et al.* (1977) compared single-point acupuncture at a single session with and without codeine with placebo 'acupuncture' with and without codeine in its effect on surgical dental pain. He found that at 30 minutes acupuncture had the greatest effect, i.e. more than codeine and placebo, and from two to three hours, acupuncture plus codeine produced significantly more analgesia than either alone.

Transcutaneous electrical nerve stimulation (TENS, TCNS, TNS)

This was first described by Hymes in 1973 for the management of acute postincisional pain. Controlled studies (Hymes *et al.* 1973, Cooperman *et al.* 1975) showed that patients receiving TENS following abdominal surgery required no medication or less postoperative analgesic medication compared to those on whom nonfunctional TENS units were applied. A similar analgesic effect was found following hip surgery (Pike 1978). This study demonstrated the apparent lack of nausea and vomiting associated with this method compared to opioid analgesia. Following herniorrhaphy, Bussey and Jackson (1981) showed a 65% reduction in the need for any supplementary medication.

The reduction in the need for analgesic medication is not so obvious in those patients who have been taking opioid medication for more than two weeks prior to surgery, and the implication is that opioid tolerance is the same as, or leads to, tolerance to TENS. The use of TENS leads to a reduction in the prevalence of pulmonary atelectasis following abdominal surgery compared to conventional opioid medication (Ali *et al*. 1981), and to smaller reductions in functional residual capacities and vital capacities.

Both somatic and visceral pain are affected, and the gastrointestinal peristaltic movements are relatively unaffected (Hymes *et al*. 1973). A side-effect is that the regional blood flow in the stimulated area is increased, such that capillary oozing may persist after hip surgery (Pike 1978). This may indicate improved capillary flow and lead to improved wound healing.

Some of the recent clinical trials have failed to show an improvement in pain relief by TENS beyond that achieved by placebo application of a mechanical device. This may merely reflect the considerable contributory effect of a powerful placebo.

Choice of systemic analgesic — opioid or non-opioid

The systemic analgesics are compared in Table 9.6. Although ketamine acts on the sigma receptor, which was originally classified as an opioid receptor, the spectrum of activity is very different from that of morphine. Clonidine and xylazine are also analgesic and can inhibit the withdrawal syndrome from morphine, but these properties are derived not from binding with an opioid receptor but from activity which converges with that of the *result* of opioid binding. However, since these latter have only been used for clinical postoperative pain experimentally and intraspinally, they have not been included in the table.

Choice of non-steroidal anti-inflammatory drug (NSAID)

The duration, route and side-effects of the commonly used NSAIDs are compared in Table 9.7. All these drugs have analgesic, antipyretic and anti-inflammatory properties. The analgesic action is due to both central and peripheral properties. They are especially effective against the pain of inflammation and trauma. At least part of this action is due to the inhibition of cyclo-oxygenase, reducing levels of prostanoids, and the interference with the synthesis of such widespread and multifunctional endogenous substances leads, inevitably, to a wide range of side-effects. They cause gastrointestinal bleeding and irritation, changes in the immune response, changes in the function of the renal, hepatic, and nervous systems, and they interfere with the processess of parturition and clotting. Gastrointestinal irritation, erosion, and bleeding is probably the most common serious side-effect and demonstrates the diversity of their actions. Salicylates, for example, are locally irritant and cause necrosis and erosions. The local effect is magnified because salicylates are absorbed through the gastric wall in a non-ionic form and ionize in the mucosal and submucosal cells, where they become trapped and accumulate to a concentration 15-20 times that of the gastric lumen. They inhibit the production of prostaglandins and increase production of leukotrienes, leading to increased gastric acid secretion and reduced blood flow. There is thus an increase in the acidity and necrosis of the gastric lining. The protective mucus secretion is inhibited, and the bleeding is prolonged because salicylates also alter the platelet cyclo-oxygenase and inhibit platelet agglutination. If given at the same time as warfarin, they increase the clotting time by competing with warfarin for the protein binding sites in plasma. Rarely, gastrointestinal bleeding may occur at low doses as a hypersensitivity response.

There is little to choose between the efficacies of the different NSAIDs. All have been shown to have equivalent efficacies to, or be better than, aspirin. The continued use of aspirin, and especially paracetamol, suggests that such 'improvements' are marginal. Some NSAIDs have been shown to be effective against visceral pain or to have a reduced ulcerogenic effect, but so far they have produced either an increased prevalence of skin rashes or have not yet achieved a widespread use.

Soluble products are less irritant to the gastric muscosa than insoluble ones and achieve absorption over a wider area and do so more quickly. Dispersible tablets are easier to swallow, especially when fluid is restricted. The propionic acids, e.g. naproxen, are better tolerated, in general, than the carboxylic acids, e.g. aspirin, but diflunisal and piroxicam are also tolerated well. Some drugs,

Table 9.6. Choice of systemic analgesic.

Drug type	Advantages	Disadvantages
Paracetamol	Reduces prostaglandin levels, especially in the brain; effective reliever of mild pain and some severe pains: pain due to bone secondaries, dysmenorrhoea	Available only by mouth or by enema. Not absorbed from stomach Not potent enough for most postoperative pain. Large doses can induce liver failure. Atopic reactions unusual but not rare
NSAIDs e.g. aspirin	Have more effect on inflammation and pain of inflammation than opioids or paracetamol. Some drugs available by injection or rectally. Cause no respiratory or cardiovascular depression	Not potent enough for pain following most visceral operations High incidence of side-effects: increased bleeding, gastric irritation, fluid retention, bronchospasm, etc.
Opioids	Capable of relieving pain of greater severity than the above, especially visceral pain; pure agonists can relieve pain of any severity if respiratory and cardiovascular depression treated Effects reversible (usually) by naloxone. Relieve anxiety. Act rapidly[1]. Available by many routes[2]	Relieve sharp pain poorly except in high dosage Cause ventilatory and cardiovascular depression in high dosage May cause ileus and urinary retention, nausea and itching
Inhalational, e.g. nitrous oxide	Effects rapid and reversible[1] Nitrous oxide interferes little with the function of the heart and lungs Patient-demand system inherently safe	Analgesic effect transient Continuous inhalation tiring and may, if gases dry, cause retrosternal soreness Equipment bulky Trichloroethylene causes nausea, tachypnoea and tachycardia.

Table 9.6. Continued.

Drug type	Advantages	Disadvantages
Ketamine	Does not depress respiration or reflexes (except by analgesia of stimulated part) Provides profound somatic analgesia	When used alone, frequently causes hallucinations and disorientation, diplopia, dizziness and drowsiness Causes an increased heart rate and blood pressure (increased cardiac work)
Nefopam	Respiratory depression very slight	Does not reliably relieve pain High incidence of side-effects: nausea, sweating, restlessness and tachycardia

Notes
1 *See* Chapter 13.
2 *See* Table 9.5.

e.g. fenbufen, sulindac, have less ulcerogenic activity than aspirin or naproxen but have a higher incidence of skin rashes. All are constipating, with the possible exception of mefenamic acid, for which diarrhoea is a toxic complication. All are anti-inflammatory, but the anti-inflammatory properties of ibuprofen and mefenamic acid are less than average.

Some are available by rectum, thereby avoiding the difficulties of oral ingestion in a patient whose laryngeal reflexes may be incompetent, although absorption from the rectal mucosa tends to be more unreliable. Some have sufficiently long durations of action (naproxen and diflunisal — 12 hours: piroxicam — 24 hours) to be given preoperatively and to be effective until full consciousness and reflexes have returned.

Side-effects are many but, with the exception of atopy, are rarely serious after one or few recommended doses.

For some somatic or inflammatory pains, they may be sufficient sole analgesia. Even for abdominal visceral pain, they are able to reduce the need for opioid or other analgesia.

Table 9.7. Comparative side-effects of some NSAIDs.

Drug (recommended maximum daily adult dose, mg)	Routes available	Duration (hours)	Side-effects
Diclofenac (150)	Oral i.m. Rectal	8 8	Painful by injection Potentiates lithium and digoxin
Diflunisal (1000)	Oral	12	Well tolerated but may cause rashes and tinnitus Potentiates warfarin and indomethacin Inhibited by aspirin
Fenbufen (900)	Oral	12	Active ingredient released by hydrolysis in the plasma, therefore less local gastric irritation, but higher risk of skin rashes and erythema multiforme Inhibited by aspirin
Fenoprofen (3000)	Oral	6	Less GI bleeding than with aspirin but more than with naproxen No increased effect with age Increased incidence of blurred vision and amblyopia Potentiates warfarin
Flurbiprofen (300)	Oral	6–8	More effective than aspirin or naproxen Increased effect with age Increased prevalence of fluid retention Potentiates warfarin; inhibits frusemide
Ibuprofen (2400)	Oral	6–8	Fewer side-effects than aspirin but less anti-inflammatory activity
Indomethacin (200)	Oral Rectal	Tablets — 8 Suppositories — 12	May cause headache, stomatitis (rectal), tenesmus, toxic hepatitis, hyperglycaemia, chest pain, alopecia, blurred vision and periorbital pain

Table 9.7. Continued.

Drug (recommended maximum daily adult dose, mg)	Routes available	Duration (hours)	Side-effects
Indomethacin *Continued*			May cause early closure of the ductus arteriosus Inhibited by aspirin, potentiates warfarin and lithium; potentiated by diflunisal; inhibits the antihypertensive effect of beta-blockers
Mefenamic acid (1500)	Oral	6–8	May cause diarrhoea because of associated proctocolitis; haemolytic anaemia and other blood dyscrasias may occur Non-oliguric renal failure also may occur
Naproxen (1000)	Oral Rectal	12	Inhibits the action of frusemide and may cause fluid retention Potentiates lithium and is potentiated by probenecid
Piroxicam (20)	Oral Rectal	>24	Fluid retention and GI bleeding have been reported more frequently than after most NSAIDs Potentiates warfarin
Sulindac (400)	Oral	12	A prodrug — no local effect on the gastric mucosa May cause diarrhoea, flatulence, gastric cramps and pruritus, alopecia, photosensitivity, erythema multiforme and toxic epidermal necrolysis, exfoliative dermatitis, cardiac failure (from fluid retention), palpitations and hypertension May discolour the urine
Tolmetin (1800)	Oral	6–8	Similar to naproxen

Choice of opioid

Opioid agonists, partial agonists, and antagonists

All opioids bind to opioid receptors, by definition. Some have a powerful maximal action, some have a less than maximal effect, and some have very little characteristic opioid effect at all. They compete for the receptor with varying degrees of affinity, and once attached the binding forces also vary with the identity of the opioid. Thus, if buprenorphine is preceded by naloxone, the naloxone is not easily displaced by the buprenorphine and will prevent the action of the latter. However, if buprenorphine precedes naloxone, the binding is too strong to allow significant displacement and antagonism by naloxone. The explanation for this may be differential affinities for different states of the mu receptor, but the practical implications are obvious.

In clinical terms, the action of a full agonist increases with the dose. Theoretically, once all the receptors have been occupied, there can be no further effect due to an increase in dose, but this stage is not reached until there is profound medullary (cardiovascular and ventilatory) depression. The partial agonists have a lower ceiling of effect, such that significant ventilatory or cardiac depression may not occur at any dose in some patients. The same is true of analgesia, so that although these drugs may be safer, they are less effective as analgesics. Furthermore, since they compete for the same binding sites as the full agonists, the simultaneous administration of drugs in both groups has an effect which is intermediate between the effect of either. There are four possibilities:

1 The patient has received large amounts of the agonist before the partial agonist: the effect of the agonist is reduced, because of competition for the receptors.
2 The patient has received large amounts of the partial agonist before the agonist is given: the effect of the agonist is reduced because of the prior occupancy of the receptors.
3 The patient has received small amounts of the agonist before the partial agonist is given.
4 The patient has received small amounts of the partial agonist before the full agonist is given.

In cases 3 and 4 further receptor occupancy will enhance the opioid effect and the effect of the two drugs will be additive.

A partial agonist is an agonist which has less effect than an full agonist. In competition with a full agonist, it is a partial antagonist. A pure antagonist has no opioid effects of its own and will antagonize the effect of a pure or partial agonist provided that it can compete for and occupy the opioid receptor.

As explained in a previous chapter, not all opioid receptors are the same, and each drug or ligand can be an agonist at one receptor, but an antagonist or partial antagonist at another. The effect of any opioid depends not only on the activity of each receptor, but also on the spectrum of activity of any other opioids acting at the same time.

The comparative prevalence of side-effects of equianalgesic doses of the established opioids shown in Table 9.8 demonstrates that, in general, the tendency to produce a feeling of well-being is accompanied by one which causes nausea and dizziness. (Most of this comparison is derived from the paper of Morrison *et al.* 1971.) There is, however, considerable individual patient variation in the response to the opioids, such that a patient who is nauseated by one opioid may not be nauseated by an equianalgesic dose of another, although both opioids have a similar overall tendency to produce nausea.

The pharmacological properties of many of the opioids are discussed and compared in Chapter 5.

Choice of oral opioid

Although levorphanol and methadone have a greater oral bio-availability than morphine, morphine elixir or tablets remains the most wisely used effective oral opioid. The action can be prolonged by the use of slow-release preparations (Duromorph) or a drug-releasing matrix (MST Continus).

Rectal preparations

Although pentazocine is available rectally, absorption is unreli-

Table 9.8. Scale effects of narcotic analgesics. A, much better than average; B, better than average; C, average; D, worse than average; E, much worse than average.

Drug and dose	Lack of sedation, tranquillity[1]	Nausea, vomiting	Dizziness, hypotension, and restlessness
Dextromoramide 5 mg	E	B	B
Diamorphine 5 mg	A	C	C
Dihydrocodeine 50 mg	D	A	A
Dihydromorphinone 2 mg	A	E	E
Dipipanone 25 mg	E	A	B
Fentanyl 0.2 mg	E	D	D
Levorphanol 2 mg	A	D	B
Methadone 10 mg	C	C	B
Morphine 10 mg	B	D	C
Oxycodone 10 mg	B	D	B
Oxymorphone 1.5 mg	A	E	E
Papaveretum 20 mg	A	C	D
Pentazocine 30 mg	D[2]	B	D
Pethidine 100 mg	B	D	E
Phenazocine 2 mg	E	B	A
Phenoperidine 2 mg	E	B	A

Notes
1 Tranquillity is assumed to be desirable, and those which cause more tranquillity are cited as 'better'.
2 Pentazocine causes confusion, hypnosis, and stupor more often than tranquillity.

able. Oxycodone when available provides analgesia for eight hours or more. Dextromoramide has a relatively short duration of action, so that morphine suppositories remain the most useful available rectal opioid.

Opioids for spinal administration

Many substances have been injected spinally for the purpose of pain relief. They have been predominantly opioids — fentanyl, pethidine, pentazocine, meptazinol, bremazocine, and buprenorphine have all been used as well as morphine and diamorphine. Droperidol has been shown to augment spinal opioid analgesia, and clonidine and xylazine have been shown to be powerfully analgesic at the spinal level. Ketamine, injected spinally, was not an effective analgesic.

The ideal spinal drug is lipid-soluble, so that it is absorbed into the cord rather than remaining in the flow of the cerebrospinal fluid. However, high lipid solubility favours uptake by the epidural fat and by the systemic perfusion of the epidural space, since the drug is absorbed through the capillary membrane as well as through the capillary pores. A smaller proportion of a lipid-soluble drug crosses the dura to reach the CSF. Lipid-soluble drugs cross membranes and enter and leave the spinal cord readily. The dose of drug required for epidural analgesia is of the same order as that required for systemic effect. The intrathecal dose is several times smaller. An exception to the rule is diamorphine: this crosses the membranes as lipid-soluble diamorphine or monoacetylmorphine, but is hydrolysed within the spinal cord to the lipid-insoluble morphine, and the duration of action is longer than would be expected from its lipid solubility. Thus, although less epidural diamorphine reaches the CSF than epidural morphine, the effect is greater, so that morphine and diamorphine are equipotent. The larger molecular weight drugs also cross the dural barrier less readily, with the exception of fentanyl and fentanyl-like drugs, which cross the dural barrier relatively easily.

Drugs which are lipid-insoluble, like morphine, are longer-lasting, because a depot of drug remains in the CSF, but that part of the drug is subject to movement of fluid and may spread towards the brain to cause delayed ventilatory depression. The greater the lipid solubility and the slower the rate of injection, the more localized is the absorption and effect.

Buprenorphine is very lipid-soluble and is very effective intrathecally. It is more effective as an analgesic epidurally than systemically, but the difference is not as great as for diamorphine (Alexander & Black 1984).

Fentanyl is very effective epidurally, but the duration of action is short and the amounts required are almost as great as for systemic administration.

Lofentanil, like buprenorphine, is very lipid-soluble and has very strong binding to the opioid receptors. Like buprenorphine, its systemic action is prolonged (>24 hours), its onset is slow, and it is not reliably reversed by naloxone. It has been shown to be superior, given epidurally, to buprenorphine, and it has a much greater, and more localized, effect when given intrathecally.

Diamorphine and lofentanil appear, therefore, to be the opioids of choice for spinal administration, but lofentanil must be used with extreme caution because of the lack of an effective antagonist and the risk of apnoea. It should be used in a small-volume injection to avoid rostral spread of drug.

Drug combinations

In practice, it is often prudent and beneficial to use a combination of analgesic drugs and methods. Elevation, immobilization, liniments, application of warmth, ultrasound, and transcutaneous nerve stimulation are analgesic manoeuvres which are frequently used in combination with analgesic drugs to improve the effect or reduce the analgesic drug requirement. A drug with secondary analgesic properties may be used to potentiate the primary analgesic rather than produce analgesia by itself. Other drugs (antiemetics, doxapram) are used to counteract the side-effects of the primary analgesics so that analgesically effective doses can be tolerated. So too can the principal analgesic drugs be combined with enhanced effect without necessarily increasing toxicity.

Opioids plus NSAIDs (or cyclo-oxygenase inhibitors)

It has been demonstrated in the care of terminal pain that very small doses of opioid can enhance remarkably the analgesic effect of NSAIDs, even in advanced cancer pain. Postoperative pain of mild to moderate severity can frequently be controlled by this drug combination, and co-proxamol is used widely. Even the pain following gastrointestinal surgery has been shown to be greatly reduced or eliminated by large doses of NSAIDs when used in an analgesic trial, and the combination of these two types of drugs can reduce the requirement of each of them.

Opioids plus local anaesthetics

Opioids reduce the expectation of pain, anxiety, fear of death and disfigurement, and are often used as concomitant medication for procedures under local anaesthesia. Postoperatively, they have been shown to prolong the effectiveness of epidural analgesia, even in low dosage. Regional opioid analgesia is often effected by the epidural application of opioid dissolved in local anaesthetic so that anaesthesia of the most painful segment is combined with analgesia of a much wider area.

Opioids plus ketamine

Given alone, postoperatively, ketamine in analgesic doses causes dysphoria, disorientation and delusions. Ketamine in low dose (e.g. 0.1 $mg^{-1} kg^{-1} hour^{-1}$) can control severe postoperative pain when combined with a moderate level of opioid which by itself is analgesically inadequate.

Summary

The routine prescription of an intramuscular opioid on patient demand for postoperative pain relief does not reflect the wide choice of drug, route, timing, method, or administrator of analgesia. In recent years, there has been a resurgence of interest in the problem of postoperative pain and the development of newer, more effective means of relieving pain. There has arisen a renewed interest in local anaesthetic procedures, in spinally applied opioids, and in the development of patient-controlled analgesia. New safer and effective drugs are being developed. However, more effective analgesia may be achieved only at the expense of greater watchfulness, more intensive nursing, or greater expenditure on equipment. The existing resources can be utilized to the full by greater understanding of the actions and duration of action of the established drugs, by combining the advantages of one drug or method with another, and by being constantly aware of the possibility and penalties of postoperative pain. One of the studies reported (Ellis *et al*. 1982) failed to confirm an improvement of pain relief by the use of patient-controlled analgesia, probably because of the high standard of staff awareness of postoperative pain and of frequency of analgesic medication.

CHAPTER 10
Regional Anaesthesia and Analgesia

Local anaesthesia can relieve all forms of postoperative pain, except those due to sensory deprivation itself, such as phantom limb pain. It may be especially indicated when other forms of analgesia are unacceptably ineffective or when their side-effects, e.g. ventilatory depression or gastric irritation, increase the postoperative risk, for example in the obese, the bronchitic and the ulcerated, or are distressing, e.g. nausea, vomiting, constipation.

To most of these patients, and to many others, local anaesthesia is an effective, acceptable, alternative form of pain relief. That it is not used more suggests that there are disadvantages, complications, and contraindications which counterbalance its obvious advantages. It is also true that regional techniques are relatively uncommon because the training in such techniques is less thorough and widespread than in general anesthesia. Suitably trained staff are not usually available throughout the postoperative period to renew the analgesia as necessary. Some of these disadvantages are considered later and are not necessarily the same as those which apply to local anaesthesia for the operative procedure. However, these latter disadvantages influence the choice between general and regional anaesthesia so that local anaesthesia may not be instituted at a time when conditions for so doing are most favourable.

Disadvantages of regional anaesthesia during surgery

1 The spread of the local anaesthetic block must extend outside the operated area to include those structures which must be retracted, packed, or pressed upon. It may cause sympathetic blockade.
2 The patient may be anxious or even embarassed at the thought of being awake during the operation. Excessive anxiety may cause the patient to react violently when touched because of the interpretation of all sensation as the expected pain.

3 Procedures may be required which are outside the operated area, such as stomach washouts, catheterization, etc.
4 The operation may have to be extended because of unexpected disease or difficulty, beyond the duration of the initial bolus of local anaesthetic.
5 Greater gaseous distension and visibility are available during laparoscopy when muscle relaxation and general anaesthesia are used than when local anaesthetic only is used.
6 The surgeon may wish to discuss the findings of the operation with junior or senior colleagues for the purposes of training, teaching, or consultation, and would not wish to alarm the patient unnecessarily while considering all the possibilities of diagnosis and implications.
7 Local anaesthesia is more variable than general anaesthesia in its extent and duration: the persistence of unblocked segments or the return of sensation would require the conversion to general anaesthesia.
8 The patient may have uncontrollable movements, such as coughing, sneezing, twitching, which are unrelated to the operation but interfere with its performance.
9 The loss of muscle tone may make the diagnosis or procedure more difficult, for example during excision of an anal fistula.

Many of these disadvantages can be overcome by combining local anaesthesia with light general anesthesia or neuroleptanalgesia. Postoperatively, the local anaesthesia can be used as the sole analgesia or used to reduce the requirement of systemic analgesia.

The term local anaesthesia is used instead of local analgesia because these drugs and techniques reduce or remove all forms of sensation and not only pain. This property has both advantages and disadvantages over other forms of pain relief.

Advantages of postoperative local anaesthesia

1 Local anaesthetics are effective against all forms of pain, sharp and dull, intermittent or crescendo, somatic and visceral. They do not just render it more tolerable: they can eliminate it altogether. Effective coughing following thoracic and abdominal operations or following multiple fractured ribs becomes possible.
2 Pain relief is accompanied by very little change of consciousness. Although local anaesthetics do have a systemic action and may

(e.g. lignocaine) cause sedation, this effect is less than with other forms of pain relief.
3 Ventilatory drive is unaltered, as is the ability to overcome airway obstruction. However, a subjective feeling of difficulty of breathing may occur (*see below*).
4 The reduction of muscle tone may be an advantage, as in the relief of pain after haemorrhoidectomy or after plastic surgery when a limb must be held in a fixed position for prolonged periods.
5 Sympathetic blockade improves blood flow by decreasing the vascular resistance. This aids perfusion following arterial reconstructive surgery. It reduces the prevalence of thromboembolism. It is indicated following accidental intra-arterial injection of thiopentone or for other causes of vasospasm such as the occasional reaction to the presence of an arterial cannula.

Disadvantages of postoperative local anaesthesia

1 Although local anaesthesia is effective pain relief, it does not counteract the expectations of death, disability, and deformity which contribute to postoperative fear and distress. Paradoxically, because the patient is pain-free, he tends to be given less reassurance unless the nursing routine includes regular enquiries.
2 Total local anaesthesia is difficult to achieve when pain and discomfort are perceived through a wide distribution of nerves. Total hysterectomy and abdominoperineal resection involve thoracic and caudal segments. Upper abdominal surgery involves the subdiaphragmatic structures, which may give rise to pain through the phrenic (cervical) nerve or to pain from the nasogastric tube via cranial nerves. Total relief of pain following thoracotomy is difficult to achieve by local anaesthetic alone when the thoracic drains are sited at the lung base and at the apex: all thoracic and some of the cervical nerves can be stimulated.
3 Local anaesthesia is often accompanied by sympathetic blockade, and when this is widespread, as in spinal (intrathecal or epidural) anaesthesia, hypotension may result. This may be severe and sudden at the initial injection or at subsequent top-up injections. If segments above the fifth thoracic are involved, the sympathetic drive to the heart is diminished and bradycardia may occur.

4 Vasodilation leads to heat loss. If severe, unpleasant feelings of cold and shivering, or hypothermia, occur.

5 Vasoconstriction is a natural compensating mechanism for fluid loss postoperatively, maintaining blood pressure, venous return, and cardiac output. If lost, these functions must be monitored and managed.

6 The loss of all sensation to a part makes it more liable to injury, in that it is unprotected by further pain, and nerve compression, pressure sores, ischaemic damage, etc. may occur. Because of the loss of proprioception, it is difficult to control, so that an anaesthetic arm may act like a flail and if covered in plaster it can do considerable harm to the rest of the body.

7 Local anaesthesia demands a level of skill and a knowledge of anatomy and pharmacology not usually consistently available in the general postoperative ward. It demands equipment, aseptic technique and adequate space in which to perform nerve blockade without interruption or disturbance, and it requires a high standard of illumination at any time that the anaesthesia must be renewed.

8 Since the patient is in pain at the times of anaesthetic renewal, it may be distressing for him to adopt the position necessary for the nerve block to be performed, or it may be difficult for him to remain motionless during the procedure.

9 Repeated nerve blockade may not be feasible because of the position, thickness or hardness of the dressing.

10 Repeated nerve block by repeated needling can be avoided by the use of cannulae inserted at the time of the operation, and sudden changes of blood pressure can be avoided by the use of continuous infusions, but such equipment, sterile packs, infusion pumps, cannulae, filters, and nerve locating devices, are expensive, and the techniquie must be advantageous if the cost is to be compared to an ampoule of morphine.

11 There are complications of this technique which are the results of local injury, migration of cannulae, injection into a site other than the perineural tissue, and of toxicity of the drugs.

Contraindications to local anaesthetic blockade

1 Sepsis at the site of injection or within the circulation.

2 Abnormal bleeding or clotting times, e.g. liver failure, anticoagulant therapy.
3 Allergy to the drugs.
4 Unwilling or frightened patient.
5 Prior insensibility of an area of proposed blockade, where nerves are subject to damage by the injecting needle, e.g. the median nerve at the wrist. The removal of the pain sensation because of either concurrent general anaesthesia or a previous nerve block removes also the warning of nerve damage or compression at the time of the injection.
6 When sensation provides an essential warning of further damage, as, for example, when an acute injury which is liable to swell is enclosed in a cast.
7 When the safety of the part cannot be ensured, for example for minor operations performed on out-patients when the anaesthetic part cannot be protected.
8 When adequate analgesia cannot be obtained without using toxic amounts of anaesthetic drug; this applies to repeat injections also. This consideration is most relevant when the area of required anaesthesia is large, when the site of injection is vascular, and when the demands for analgesia are frequent.
9 Ignorance and inability to treat the complications of local anaesthesia.

Complications of local anaesthesia

Complications may be relevant to a specific local anaesthetic block or relevant to local anaesthetic blockade in general. The non-specific complications are related to injury caused by the injecting needle or cannula, or to the action of the drug at or around the site of the nerve block, or to a combination of the two.

Local complications

Local anaesthetic solutions cause changes in the cell membranes of nerves and other structures: they can cause vasodilation or vasoconstriction and alter the local pH of the tissues. Most are toxic to skeletal muscle and can cause, usually reversibly, rhabdomyolysis.

Nerve damage

Needles may puncture the nerve axons and sheath, inducing neurofibrillary growth and an abnormal sense organ at the site of damage. This causes local tenderness, abnormal pain appearing to arise from a more distal site, a continuous pain, and one that is influenced by the level of circulating catecholamines. Nerves may be damaged by the local toxicity of strong local anaesthetic solutions. This was more common when crystals of amethocaine were used for subarachnoid anaesthesia; incomplete dissolution led to the nerves being exposed to very high concentrations of the drug and to local or regional nerve palsies. Even 5% lignocaine is associated with pain on injection and incomplete recovery of the nerve conduction. Where cocaine is used for surface analgesia of the cornea, the ischaemia caused by the associated vasoconstriction can lead to pitting of the surface.

Nerves may be damaged by injection of solutions into the neurovascular sheath below a non-distensible retinaculum or within rigid compartments, and the pressure of the injection may cause reversible or non-reversible axonal changes. Sites of increased risk are those of the median nerve below the flexor retinaculum at the wrist, that of the ulnar nerve where it lies in the groove of the humerus, that of the common peroneal nerve as it lies on the neck of the fibula, and that of the infraorbital nerve within the infraorbital canal. Nerve damage may also be caused by puncture of a blood vessel with haematoma formation, for example within the spinal canal or retroperitoneally during coeliac plexus block.

Vascular complications

Blood vessels are not uncommonly punctured or cannulated during nerve blockade. This complication is not usually serious, except when it causes nerve pressure or when the clotting mechanism is defective. Intravascular injection may result in a toxic plasma level of the local anaesthetic or of the vasoconstrictor which may accompany it. Vasoconstrictors may cause profound ischaemia when injected into or around small arteries and are contraindicated in nerve blocks of the fingers, toes, and penis. Accidental injection into a cerebral artery during stellate ganglion block or field block of the tonsils could cause convulsions and unconsciousness after, say, only 0.2 ml of lignocaine 1%. Accidental puncture of the aorta and inferior vena cava can occur during lumbar sympathetic or coeliac plexus block. Bleeding within the coats of the aorta could cause a dissecting aneurysm, and damage to the wall of the vena cava could form the locus of a thrombus which may later cause a pulmonary embolus. Considerable bleeding may occur from either vessel, and adequate compression can rarely be applied to them.

Haemorrhage within the spinal canal may lead to compression of the cord and also to fibrosis, so that on subsequent occasions the irregular spread of the local anaesthetic would lead to patchy anaesthesia. Puncture of the thoracolumbar anterior spinal artery, or constriction because of the use of vasoconstrictors, may lead to ischaemia of the entire lumbar section of the cord. Anterior spinal artery ischaemia leads predominantly to a loss of motor power or to dissociated sensory loss, because the damage is primarily in the anterior part of the cord. The incidence of damage is reduced by epidural puncture below the third lumbar vertebra.

Haematomata may also form a culture medium for infection, and abscesses, although rare, are more likely following vascular damage. Subperiosteal haematomata can lead to new bone formation and structural damage.

Infection

Injection through infected skin or tissues carries the infection more deeply, A hollow needle may carry a cylinder of tissue to the deeper structures. Where bacteraemia already exists, tissue damage or haemorrhage may localize the infection to form an abscess. The vasodilation caused by strong solutions of local anaesthetics or by the accompanying sympathetic blockade may overcome the body's natural barrier to bacterial or fungal invasion and spread the infection. Regional anaesthesia is associated with inhibition of leucocyte aggregation and adherence of leucocytes to the intima of blood vessels. The significance of this is unknown (Wall 1984).

Local tissue irritation

Swelling, cellulitis, and sloughing may also occur because of chemical contamination of the solution or apparatus of nerve blockade. Some local anaesthetics can release the nickel and zinc from metal instruments or even from synthetic rubber stoppers that contain excessive zinc oxide. Superficial sloughing may follow a large skin wheal when vasoconstrictors are used.

Damage to adjacent structures

The pleura may be damaged during brachial plexus block, intercostal nerve block, stellate ganglion block, thoracic sympathetic or paravertebral nerve block, or coeliac plexus block. Provided that only the pleura is entered and fluid-filled syringes are attached to the needles at the time, the puncture is of little consequence. If the lung is punctured also, gas leaks from the lung into the pleura and a pneumothorax forms. The leak is often accompanied by pain, but if a small-bore needle is used the puncture usually heals spontaneously. If the needle is of large bore, if the patient has emphysema or bronchospasm, if the leak occurred during mechanical ventilation, or if the patient exercises soon afterwards, a large pneumothorax or a tension pneumothorax forms. This causes collapse of the affected lung and, if there is a tension pneumothorax, a chest drain with an underwater seal is required. A tension pneumothorax may develop very quickly and be life-threatening. (A chest drain should always be available wherever these procedures are performed.) Sometimes, the pneumothorax develops very slowly and may not be apparent on radiographs taken soon after the needle puncture.

Bradycardia

This may be due to depression of the myocardium (*see below*) or be due to blockade of the cardioaccelerator nerves from sympathetic blockade of the first four thoracic segments or the cervical sympathetic chain. Although cervical sympathetic block can relieve the pain of an acute myocardial infarction, it may be accompanied by a lethal bradycardia.

Fainting

Psychogenically induced cardiovascular collapse is most commonly seen in the dental chair or prior to otorhinolaryngological procedures. It is probably due to the anxiety some patients feel before this form of surgery. The pain and fear cause pallor, nausea, cold sweating, and a sudden fall of blood pressure. Cerebral hypoxia with loss of consciousness may occur at the time of the insertion of the needle or at the time of the injection of the local anaesthetic. In the latter case, it may be due, in whole or in part, to the rapid absorption of the drug from the tissues of the head and neck which are relatively vascular, especially when inflamed. In either case, hypoxic tremors and convulsions may occur before the patient can be placed in a horizontal position. The cardiovascular collapse also causes a larger than normal proportion of the drug in the plasma to be distributed to the best-perfused organs such as the heart and the brain.

Changes in intracranial pressure

Extradural injection of local anaesthetic or any other solution causes a rise in intracranial pressure. This rise varies directly with the amount of the solution and the speed of the injection and inversely with the size of the intervertebral foramina and the intracranial compliance (Hilt *et al.* 1986). It should be used with extreme caution, if at all, in those with intracranial hypertension or a space-occupying lesion, and in these patients accidental dural puncture can produce intracranial haemorrhage, medullary coning, and death.

Toxicity

Toxicity of local anaesthetics may be due to an absolute overdose in a normally susceptible individual, a normal dose in an abnormally susceptible patient, accidental intravenous or intra-arterial injection, or rapid absorption from a vascular site or from inflamed tissues. Toxicity will be increased when biotransformation and excretion of the drug is reduced, in conditions of acidosis, when the cardiac output is reduced, when plasma protein binding is low, and when the organs under consideration are already damaged or diseased. It can be reduced by the use of vasoconstrictors such as adrenaline and felypressin, which reduce the rate of systemic absorption but have a danger and toxicity of their own (*see above*).

Diagnosis of toxicity

In heavy, but non-toxic, dosages lignocaine, prilocaine, and procaine cause sleepiness and general anaesthesia — a sign of central nervous system depression. In toxic doses, central nervous system stimulation is apparent. The signs of increasing toxicity are:
1 Restlessness.
2 Light-headedness.
3 Numbness of the tongue and lips.
4 Visual disturbance, e.g. dimness, blurring, or even double vision.
5 Heaviness of limbs or trunk.
6 Bupivacaine may cause ventricular extrasystoles.
(At this stage, hearing is usually well preserved.)
7 Muscular twitching.
8 Unconsciousness.
9 Generalized convulsions.
10 Respiratory arrest.
11 Non-postural hypotension.
12 Asystole.

If the intravenous bolus is rapid, cardiovascular symptoms of tachycardia and extrasystoles, hypotension, and arrest may predominate to the exclusion of the others. If accidental injection into a cerebral artery occurs during stellate ganglion injection or during a tonsillar bed field block, convulsions, coma and respiratory arrest may be the first signs of toxicity.

There may be an abnormality of taste (allogneusis or hypogneusis), but this is not a constant finding.

At increasing concentrations, the level of consciousness falls, but it is a consistent finding that the sense of hearing is relatively spared so that the patient must be assured that treatment is available for this complication and has been started. However, many of these signs may occur from other causes. Accidental subdural or intrathecal injection can cause a feeling of heaviness of the chest and a difficulty in breathing, although, objectively, the tidal and minute ventilation can be normal. Shivering and shaking from cold may be mistaken for muscular twitching and may occur in the unpremedicated patient with extensive sympathetic blockade and vasodilation. The heat loss causes shivering or shaking in the unanaesthetized parts of the body. Agitation or restlessness can be caused by the adrenaline which may accompany the local anaesthetic, or by ephedrine which may be given for hypotension.

Treatment of toxicity

Treatment of toxicity should be directed towards maintenance of oxygenation of the tissues, especially the brain, the oxygen consumption of which can be very large during convulsions. The airway should be established or maintained, ventilation may have to be assisted mechanically, and it should be enriched with oxygen. The cardiac output may have to be increased by increasing venous return, adjusting the rate and increasing the force of contraction. The venous return should be increased quickly by tipping the patient head-down (unless a dose of hyperbaric local anaesthetic or spinal opioid has just been administered), by infusion of fluids, and by the use of a vasoconstrictor. If adrenaline or ephedrine is used, this will increase the force of contraction of the heart also. Atropine and ephedrine are used to remedy bradycardia. If cardiac arrest occurs, closed-chest cardiac message is usually effective in maintaining the cardiac output and enabling redistribution of the drug. The protein binding and degree of ionization of etidocaine and bupivacaine at pH 7.4 are greater than those of lignocaine and prilocaine, and resuscitative measures will need to be prolonged. The cardiotoxic effects of bupivacaine can be treated successfully in animals with large doses of adrenaline and atropine, with the addition of verapamil where necessary (R. Lundh, personal communication).

The muscular twitching and convulsions should be controlled with an anticonvulsant such as diazepam emulsion (10–12 mg), which causes less cardiovascular depression than thiopentone. Conversely, thiopentone works more quickly and can be given cautiously while waiting for the diazepam to take effect in a rapidly deteriorating situation. Suxamethonium controls the twitching in the muscles but does not affect the convulsant activity of the brain, and should be used only as an aid to intubation where this is necessary to maintain adequate ventilation (*see also* Table 10.2).

Atopy

Hypersensitivity or allergic reaction to drugs of the amide group (e.g. lignocaine) is extremely rare. It occurs more commonly with drugs of the ester group (e.g. tetracaine), which are now rarely used in the postoperative period, or with the preservative methylhydroxybenzoate which is found in the multidose vial. Allergic reactions present as peripheral vasoconstriction, bronchospasm, oedema, and cardiovascular collapse. They are treated, as elsewhere, with dilute adrenaline, fluid infusions, followed by high-dose steroid, and antihistamines to modify the subsequent urticaria.

Avoidance of complications

A carefully taken history and examination should exclude anticoagulant therapy, allergy, psychogenic syncope, infection, and pre-existing neural damage, etc. Venous access should be secured with an indwelling venous catheter, and if hypotension is probable it can be avoided or reduced by preloading the circulation with 500–1000 ml of fluid, colloid or crystalloid. Sudden complications such as fainting or vomiting cannot be managed by a single operator, and an assistant, a tipping trolley or bed, and suction apparatus are essential. Other resuscitative equipment and drugs should be immediately available (Table 10.2).

The amount and concentration of the drug should not exceed the least effective for the nerve block, for example infiltration anaesthesia is effective with drugs in low concentrations, e.g. lignocaine 0.5%. Absorption can be delayed in some cases by the use of vasoconstrictor agents in low concentrations e.g. adrenaline 1:400000, although the peak blood levels of the fat-soluble drugs, bupivacaine and etidocaine, given into the epidural space, are little affected by the addition of vasoconstrictors. Vasoconstrictors should not be used in parts which are supplied by end-arteries, e.g. fingers and toes. They should not be used in high concentration to form the skin wheal.

Neural damage can be reduced by the use of short-bevel needles and electrical stimulation of the needle to locate the nerve. Paraesthesia while attempting to locate the nerve may be a sign of nerve damage.

Choice of local anaesthetic

Bupivacaine is the preferred agent in most cases, postoperatively, because of its long duration of action, its lesser tendency to tachyphylaxis, and because it has a high sensory:motor blockade ratio. It is less toxic than other long-acting drugs like tetracaine and amethocaine. A shorter acting drug such as lignocaine or chloroprocaine may be chosen when the speed of onset is most important.

The action of most short-acting agents can be prolonged by the addition of dilute adrenaline, but this has less effect on the lipid-soluble bupivacaine and etidocaine, whose long duration of action depends upon the amount which is stored in the myelin sheaths and the lipids of the perineural tissues. However, the action of bupivacaine can be prolonged in the intercostal space by the addition of both adrenaline and high molecular weight dextran (Simpson *et al.* 1982) (Table 10.1).

Table 10.1. Onset, duration and relative motor: sensory block of the commonly used local anaesthetics.

Drug		Onset (minutes)	Duration (hours)	Motor:sensory block approximately
Chloroprocaine	2%	10	0.5−1.5	0.2
Lignocaine	2%	10−15	1−3	0.2
Mepivacaine	2%	15	1−3	?
Bupivacaine	0.25%	15−30	3−5	0.12
Bupivacaine	0.5%	15−30	3−6	0.28
Etidocaine	1%	12	3−6	1.1

NB The duration depends upon the dose of drug injected, and the onset depends on the concentration and the site of injection. The above figures are representative only.

Choice of volume and concentration of local anaesthetic agent

This is considered under epidural nerve block.

Nerve blockade for postoperative pain relief

Although all forms of operative nerve blockade are designed to outlast the duration of the surgery, some are relatively ineffective for *postoperative* pain relief. Examples are intravenous regional anaesthesia, where release of the tourniquet is followed by dissipation of the local anaesthetic from the operated tissues, and field blocks of vascular areas which are relatively short-lasting.

Other techniques *are* suitable:
1 Long-acting local anaesthetic solutions applied before, during, or after the operation.
2 Cryothermy or neurolysis, giving more prolonged sensory loss.
3 Cannulation before or during the operation so that the effect of the local anaesthetic can be prolonged without the discomfort and risks of repeated perineural injections.
4 Nerve blocks which can be performed postoperatively with little discomfort and without infringing the safety limits of the postoperative situation.

Local anaesthetics are not uncommonly injected intraoperatively, but the opportunity to relieve pain in the early postoperative period is often wasted. Local anaesthetics can be given in combination with a vasoconstrictor and infiltrated to facilitate dissection in the operations of haemorrhoidectomy and vaginal repairs. They can be infiltrated into the skin edge prior to closure of a mastectomy incision. They can be injected into the sciatic nerve at the time of amputation of the leg, and neurolytic solutions can be applied to the coeliac ganglia at the time of pancreatectomy for malignant disease. Cryothermy can be applied to the intercostal nerves, and cannulae can be implanted between muscle layers to relieve most wound pains. The possibilities are almost endless, and most are very rewarding for the patient.

The most common and the most useful pre- and intraoperative technique for postoperative analgesia is cannulation.

Cannulation

Cannulation of the perineural spaces is feasible whenever the nerve lies in a well-defined fibrous or bony channel. It is possible in other sites, such as between muscle planes, but the cannula is likely to migrate, and repeated neural blockade becomes unreliable. Epidural cannulation is used most frequently, and despite its obvious advantage of greater analgesic efficacy than, say, systemic narcotic analgesics it is not used routinely in the general surgical ward because of the lability of blood pressure and the loss of function that it causes. It is used routinely in intensive therapy units, in cases of multiple fractured ribs, and in combination with epidural opioids. The sudden fall in blood pressure and the need for frequent monitoring can be reduced by the use of *infusion* pumps or syringes.

Advantages of infusions

1 Changes in blood pressure or loss of sensation and motor power occur gradually, such that the venous return may be maintained by infusions, drugs, or the patient's own homeostatic mechanisms as they occur.
2 The speed of the syringe and/or the concentration of the agent can be adjusted to the patient's response.
3 The need for top-ups is reduced or eliminated, and patients need not remain in pain while a member of the medical staff is called away from other commitments.
4 The constant infusion further discourages fibrin deposition on the end of the cannula so that the method can remain functional for long periods.
5 The intensity of monitoring following top-ups is disruptive of the patient's rest or sleep and may, thereby, decrease the pain tolerance.

Disadvantages of infusions

1 Continuous anaesthesia and loss of function gives rise to problems which are not so apparent when sensation, pain, and motor power are allowed to return intermittently.
2 The bladder may become distended and atonic because of lack of sensation or loss of the ability to initiate micturition.
3 Prolonged immobility of the legs and pelvic muscles increases the likelihood of deep vein thrombosis.

Cannulation of a nerve sheath

Many large nerves are surrounded by a thick fibrous sheath which protects them from damage and the shearing stress of the surrounding muscles, especially in the limbs. Some nerves are accompanied by large arteries and veins; some are invested closely by the sheath, which may contain only a small artery to the nerve itself, e.g. sciatic nerve. When the sheath contains a vein, it is lax or distensible and may be cannulated. Examples are the brachial plexus, the femoral neurovascular bundle at the inguinal ligament and the intercostal space.

Cannulation demands the use of a relatively large cannula-introducing needle which is capable of causing serious nerve damage and incomplete recovery if it penetrates the nerve itself. It is recommended that the neurovascular sheath be distended with fluid *before* introduction of the Tuohy or Crawford needle.

Cannulation of the operative wound

Local application of anaesthetic solution to abdominal wounds has been found to be an effective method of postoperative pain control, and no unwanted side-effects have been found in recent studies (Hashemi & Middleton 1983, Thomas *et al.* 1983), although the theoretical effects of delayed wound healing (Morris & Tracey 1977) were not assessed. Cannulation of either the intermuscular layer (between the internal oblique and transversus abdominis muscles) or the subcutaneous layer is effective. The cannulae used have been 'Redivac' drains, 16 gauge epidural cannulae, or perforated silastic tubing. The wound should be protected by the use of a bacterial filter, and the cannulae should be closed at the distal end to allow even irrigation from the side holes. Even so, the irrigation of the wound is very dependent on the size and position of these side holes. Possible disadvantages include the dilution of the coagulum necessary to wound healing, and inflammation because of the presence of a foreign body, albeit as inert as any suture material. Subcutaneous anaesthesia of the wound does not prevent the reflex muscle spasm which may accompany visceral pain. The method is not new (Lewis & Thomson 1953), but the more recent introduction of bacterial filters and non-reactive cannulae may make it more acceptable (Table 10.2).

Local anaesthetic techniques for postoperative pain

Spinal or peripheral nerve block?

Spinal (epidural, subdural, or subarachnoid) nerve block can relieve the pain not only of the body shell — the skin, muscle, and bone — but also of the viscera. It is suitable for the pain following a wide range of operations. The epidural space can be identified and cannulated. Local anaesthetics or opioids can be applied to this space intermittently or continuously. Conversely, spinal anaesthesia may cause sympathetic blockade and lability of the blood pressure, especially with changes of posture, and loss of heat from vasodilation, and it may cause considerable loss of function. The consequences of bleeding or infection around the nerves are more serious than with intercostal or peripheral nerve blockade.

Subarachnoid or epidural nerve block?

Subdural block is rarely attempted because of the greater technical difficulty and few, if any, advantages for postoperative pain relief.

Subarachnoid anaesthesia: advantages

1 Potent motor and sensory block.
2 Small mass of drug used and systemic toxicity unlikely.
3 Lateralization of effect possible.
4 Tachyphylaxis unlikely.
5 Rapid onset of effect.

Subarachnoid anaesthesia: disadvantages

1 Introduction of infection or contaminated material has serious consequences, such as meningitis, brain abscesses, or nerve palsies.
2 Mechanical or chemical trauma to nerves may cause permanent damage.
3 Trauma to meninges may cause adhesive arachnoiditis.
4 Trauma to blood vessels may cause ischaemia of the cord.
5 Low-pressure headaches may result: even the use of 26 or 27 gauge needles results in headache in one of every thousand punctures.
6 Too rapid injection or barbotage can lead to vacuolation and permanent damage of the nerves.
7 Sympathetic blockade, vasodilation, postural hypotension, loss of heat and urinary retention are common.

Table 10.2. Requirements for local anaesthetic procedures.

Basic equipment pack
Tipping bed or trolley
Good lighting
Facilities for washing
Gown and gloves for operator
Skin disinfectant (in galley-pot or spray), swabs and swab-holder
Sterile towels
Small hypodermic needle for anaesthetizing the superficial tissues
Dilute local anaesthetic for the superficial tissues

Equipment for resuscitation
Tipping bed or trolley
Blood pressure measurement
Suction generator and tubing
Trained and informed assistant
Intravenous cannula or infusion inserted
Nasal and oral airways
Face mask
Endotracheal tube and laryngoscope
Mechanical bellows and inflating bag (e.g. Air Viva)
A source of oxygen
Thoracic drainage trocar and cannula; underwater drains may be required when intercostal, throracic sympathetic or brachial plexus blocks are performed

Drugs for resuscitation
A vasopressor, e.g. ephedrine
Adrenaline for treatment of shock and to oppose the effects of local anaesthetic agents on the heart,
Atropine to reduce unopposed vagal stimulation
Calcium injection to reduce the effect of the local anaesthetic and to increase the cardiac tone
Steroids in large doses for treatment of shock and atopy
Diazepam emulsion *or* thiopentone for the treatment of the cerebral stimulation (tremors and convulsions)
Suxamethonium to facilitate intubation

Equipment for epidural cannulation
Basic pack
Drugs and equipment for resuscitation
Long hypodermic needle for injection of anaesthetic down to the supraspinous ligament or lamina
Scalpel blade for incision of the skin
Tuohy or Crawford needle
Device for detecting the epidural space:
a Hanging drop
b Odom's or Brook's indicator

Table 10.2. *Continued*

c Mackintosh syringe or pressure bulb.
d Glass syringe or high-quality plastic syringe for loss of resistance technique
Epidural cannula to fit the Tuohy or Crawford needle
Small-pore bacterial filter
Microporous waterproof dressing

Brachial plexus cannulation
Basic pack
Resuscitative equipment and drugs
Short, short-bevelled needle with integral cannula for piercing and filling the neurovascular sheath
Crawford-type needle: this should be blunt to avoid damage to the plexus and should be inserted into an already-distended neurovascular sheath
Cannula to pass through the above
Small-pore bacterial filter
Waterproof microporous dressing

Lumbar sympathetic and coeliac plexus block
Basic pack
Resuscitative drugs and equipment
Patients may be hypotensive following coeliac plexus block, and the intravenous cannula should be of sufficient calibre that fluids can be infused rapidly; a pre-load of 500–1000 ml is advisable
Skin marking pen
Long, fine needles for infiltration of anaesthetic down to the periosteum
Two to three 15 cm needles with stilettes, 20 gauge for location of the sympathetic chain or ganglia
Rubber discs for marking the depth of the needles
Glass syringes for loss of resistance location of the correct plane
Extension cannula to allow injection out of the beam of the X-ray
Radio-opaque contrast medium
Biplanar radioimaging
Local anaesthetic agent
Neurolytic solution if used
NB Not all plastic cannulae are compatible with the injection of alcohol

Regional anaesthetic block
Basic pack
Drugs and equipment for resuscitation
Short-bevelled needle of appropriate length with stilette *or*
Insulated needle with attached low-capacity cannula (e.g. Top-pole needle)
A nerve stimulator increases the accuracy of nerve location and the success of the nerve block
Local anaesthetic agent

8 Cannulation of the subarachnoid space is possible, but carries a greater risk of headache and infection and is rare in clinical postoperative practice.

Epidural nerve block: advantages

1 Anaesthesia more easily prolonged by cannulation.
2 Dura mater not punctured, so that CSF leak and low-pressure headache should not accompany procedure.
3 Spread of anaesthesia less affected by posture, and drug can be injected with regard to the postural requirements of the patient.

Epidural nerve block: disadvantages

1 Requires greater skill than subarachnoid puncture.
2 Larger mass of drug used so that systemic toxicity more likely, especially after repeated administration when tachyphylaxis of anaesthetic effect common.
3 Infection still common after prolonged cannulation and should be prevented by millipore filters, subcutaneous tunnelling, and possibly prophylactic antibiotics.

Epidural, extradural, or peridural nerve block?

Anatomy

The spinal cord is covered by three layers of meninges:
1 The pia mater, which invests the cord intimately.
2 The arachnoid mater, a delicate membrane which is separated from the pia by the cerebrospinal fluid.
3 The dura mater, a tough fibrous coat 'separated' from the arachnoid only by a potential space.
Outside the dura is a space filled with fibres and fat, blood vessels, lymphatics, and nerves which are still within their dural sheaths. Anteriorly are the bodies of the vertebrae, laterally are the pedicles and the intervertebral foramina, posteriorly are the spines and laminae of the vertebrae and the tough, slightly elastic ligamentum flavum. The space is deepest in the midline and in the lumbar spine, except at the lowest lumbar space, which is occupied by part of the lumbosacral plexus and, in the upright position, by the bulging of the meninges under the hydrostatic pressure of the

cerebrospinal fluid. The blood vessels lie lateral to the midline. The veins drain into the lumbar or thoracic azygos veins and hemiazygos veins, and thence into the venae cavae. They may be distended by straining, coughing, by pregnancy, and by abdominal tumours.

Technique of thoracic epidural puncture

The usual precautions of sterility and safety, e.g. tipping trolley, venous access, etc., are taken. In the mid-thoracic region, successful puncture is more certain with the paramedian (paraspinous) approach. The patient lies horizontally on his side and a skin wheal is raised 1 cm lateral to the spine of the vertebra. At this level, the tip of the vertebra lies posterior to the body of the next, inferior, vertebra. The subcutaneous tissues are anaesthetized down to the lamina. The epidural needle is introduced in the patient's horizontal plane and at 15° to the sagittal plane (Fig. 10.1). The lamina is struck and the needle is redirected more rostrally until the edge of the lamina is found. The tip of the needle is advanced into the ligamentum flavum and the stilette is withdrawn. There are many methods of locating the epidural space, but the 'loss of resistance' method is the most usual. A smoothly running syringe is half-filled with air and attached to the hub of the needle. With the syringe plunger rebounding on gentle, continuously intermittent pressure, and with counter-pressure exerted on the barrel, the needle is advanced slowly and delicately until the pressure on the plunger causes injection of air with almost no resistance. If cannulation is planned, a Tuohy needle should be used, the bevel of which should be inserted in the line of the fibres of the ligament and then turned through 90° without further advancement prior to the insertion of the cannula.

Other methods of locating the epidural space

1 Loss of resistance with fluid, usually saline.
2 The hanging drop placed on the hub of the needle which is drawn in by the subatmospheric pressure of the epidural space; this is more reliable if the patient is sitting.
3 Movement of a bubble within Odom's or Brook's indicator.

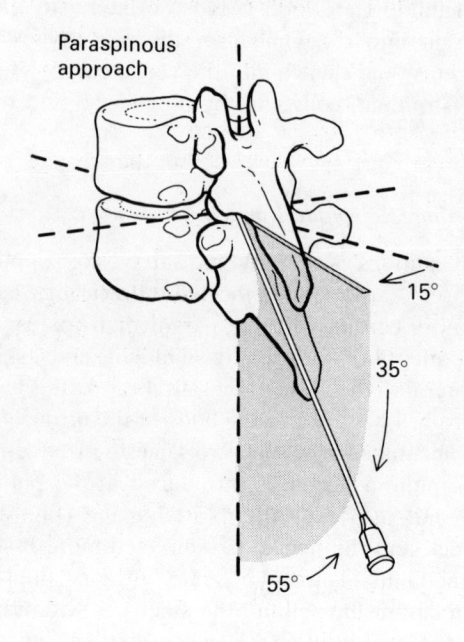

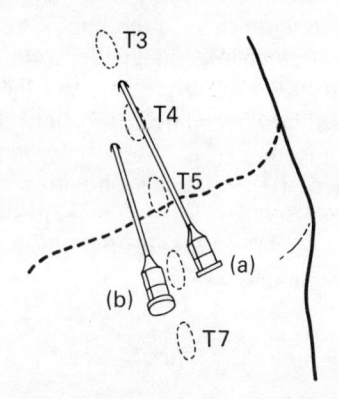

Fig. 10.1 Reproduced with permission from Cousins M. & Bridenbaugh P.O. (1980) *Neural Blockade in Clinical Anaesthesia and Management of Pain.* J.B. Lippincott Co., Philadelphia.

4 Mackintosh's indicator, which is a small air-filled rubber balloon attached to an adaptor (the balloon is filled with air when the needle lies in the ligament and the air is released when the epidural space is entered).
5 Mackintosh's spring-loaded syringe.
6 An electromanometer which shows the change in pressure when the space is entered.

Rate of injection should be slow: rapid injection causes patchy analgesia and may cause pain and neural damage by transient but excessive pressure. *Initial injection* should not exceed 3−4 ml of local anaesthetic solution. If the subarachnoid or subdural space has been entered, the extent of the nerve block will exceed expectations. It is possible for epidural and subdural or subarachnoid injections to occur simultaneously.

If dural or vascular puncture occurs, CSF or blood will probably issue from the needle. Leave the needle or cannula *in situ* and replace the stilette to reduce the fluid loss. Repeat the epidural puncture and cannulation at a different vertebral level and introduce local anaesthetic solution cautiously, since some subdural or subarachnoid leakage may occur. Withdraw the first needle or cannula.

Loss of CSF causes headache, which is worse on sitting or standing and is improved by lying down. The patient should be given plenty of fluids and simple analgesics and encouraged to lie prone. An infusion of fluid, e.g. saline, into the epidural space reduces the CSF leak, but if the epidural pressure exceeds the subarachnoid pressure, the fluid will pass into the subarachnoid space. Because the pressure varies with time, the fluids may pass intermittently in either direction.

If the headache persists, *an autologous blood patch* may be used. This requires two operators: both should scrub and don full theatre dress including hat, mask, gown, and gloves. The first operator inserts an indwelling cannula into a large vein under full aseptic conditions. The cannula is cleared of blood. The second operator inserts a needle into the epidural space close to the site of the dural puncture. Twenty millilitres of blood is withdrawn and injected slowly into the epidural space. There may be transient discomfort or paraesthesia if the blood is injected too rapidly. The patient is maintained in a horizontal position until the blood has had time to form a firm clot. Relief of headache is rapid.

Choice of volume and concentration of local anaesthetic agent

The *toxicity* of the local anaesthetic agent is related to the amount of drug absorbed by the systemic circulation. The *effectiveness* is related to the amount taken up by the neural tissues (membranes, receptors and neural stores). Both are proportional to the *mass* — the product of the volume and the concentration — of drug administered. For a given dose of drug, the slow uptake of a weak concentration (owing to a low concentration gradient) is compensated for by a larger volume being absorbed over a larger area. The *overall* onset, duration, and depth of sensory and motor block are more dependent on the identity and mass of the drug than on any other factor.

The amount of lipid-soluble drug, e.g. bupivacaine, which is stored in the myelin sheaths and fibrofatty tissue of the epidural space depends also on the amount administered. Once these stores are saturated, subsequent top-ups or infusions of the drug increase solely the concentration gradient for neural blockade or systemic absorption. If these stores have not been saturated, or have been allowed to become depleted, part of subsequent doses will dissolve in these tissues and only part will contribute to the concentration gradient and neural blockade. It follows, therefore, that the effectiveness of top-ups and infusions depends upon the previous administrations of drug and whether the nerve blockade is being maintained or re-established.

The epidural space may be considered as a cylinder of neural tissue, and the *spread* of neural block is dependent both on the *volume* of local anaesthetic solution and on the mass of drug. For example, 30 ml of 1% lignocaine injected into the lumbar epidural space achieves analgesia of dermatomes four vertebral segments higher than does 10 ml of 3% lignocaine. However, Bromage *et al.* (1964) showed that the relationship between dose and segmental spread of nerve blockade was constant for concentrations of lignocaine between 2 and 5%. Analgesia wanes because (a) drug is taken up by the systemic circulation and the concentration in the nerve membrane/channel falls, and (b) part of the volume of the initial injectate is lost through the intervertebral foramina. The anaesthesia wears off more quickly at the periphery of the area of anaesthesia and, although further administration of a small volume of concentrated drug would eventually restore the concentration at this site by diffusion, this may be so slow as to be ineffective. At least one study has demonstrated the inability of 1% bupivacaine infusions to maintain effective postoperative analgesia although the total mass administered was similar to effective regimens. The restoration of the volume of the drug maintains the anaesthesia more quickly, evenly and effectively. Despite the study mentioned above (Bromage et al. 1964), the concensus of opinion is that a low-volume, high-concentration infusion maintains a narrower band of anaesthesia than does a high-volume, low-concentration one.

The spread of analgesia is also determined by the age of the patient (on average, 2.5 ml of lignocaine 1% is required to block each vertebral segment of a 20-year-old patient, but only 1 ml is required for a patient aged 80). The intervertebral discs become thinner with age so that the intervertebral foramina become smaller and the vertebral column becomes shorter. A larger than expected spread may also occur in those patients with prolapsed discs or ankylosis, or in those who have had discs removed or vertebrae fused. It is determined by the calibre of the neural canal, which may vary considerably, by the height of the patient, and by the amount of venous distension and other space-occupying lesions of the spinal canal.

The maximal concentration of any local anaesthetic solution that should be injected is determined by dividing the subtoxic amount of local anaesthetic by the volume that is required to achieve the desired spread of anaesthesia.

The spread of analgesia that is required postoperatively depends upon the distribution of the pain and the site of injection of drug.

Optimal spread of analgesia

The distribution of analgesia should match, as far as is possible, the distribution of the pain. However, disadvantages such as loss of function as a consequence of total pain relief with consequent immobility, bladder catheterization, reduction of breathing capacity or profound postural hypotension may modify this goal to one of compromise with that which can be feasibly monitored and nursed within the facilities available. Some visceral pain, e.g. that of the lower oesophagus, can be eliminated only by risking hypotension and bradycardia. Lower abdominal pain which entails loss of use of the lower limbs and bladder risks venous thrombosis and urinary infection. Effective analgesia with fewer side-effects can be achieved by anaesthesia of the wound and visceral analgesia by systemic or, better still, epidural opioids used in combination. Wound anaesthesia can be achieved by nerve blockade of relatively few segments and, even when the sympathetic supply to the foregut is involved, compensatory vasoconstriction of other segments, constriction of the gut, and endogenously released catecholamines combine to reduce or prevent significant postural hypotension. If the rest of the body is to remain unaffected by the anaesthetic, the catheter should be sited at the most appropriate level for the postoperative pain.

Choice of site of catheter tip

The technique of epidural puncture is usually taught to the uninitiated below the second lumbar intervertebral space so that the risk of piercing the spinal cord in the adult is very small. The risk of cord damage remains a consideration in the awake labouring patient who may have great difficulty in staying still during uterine contractions. However, it is not the most appropriate site for upper or lower abdominal operations and, when the anaesthetist has achieved competence in lumbar epidural puncture, thoracic puncture should be learnt.

Abdominal operations may cause pain in segments from the fifth thoracic to the first lumbar (upper abdomen, T5–T12: lower abdomen, T7–L1) and anaesthesia on the horizontal operating table can be best achieved by siting the catheter tip midway between these vertebral levels, since the solution spreads rostrally and caudally with almost equal ease. Following operation, the pain from the wound is likely to be less extensive, say involving the dermatomes of T7–T11 only for an upper abdominal midline wound, and the degree of sensory and motor block is not required to be as complete as for surgery. However, the patient is nursed, predominantly, in a semirecumbent position, and injected solutions may be distributed differently. It is a common finding that the segments below the site of injection are more easily blocked than those above, as though the anaesthesia is influenced by gravity. In obstetric anaesthesia, this feature is utilized when the patient is rotated to remedy lateralization of the anaesthesia or by topping-up in the sitting position to achieve perineal anaesthesia. Green and Dawkins (1966) recommended that the catheter tip should be sited in the uppermost segments of the distribution of pain for epidural infusions in the sitting position. The site of the catheter is required to be less exact when top-up boluses are used, since the spread of analgesia can also be controlled by the volume of injection or by adjusting the position of the patient during the injection (and binding) of the anaesthetic agent.

Despite these observations in clinical practice, epidurograph studies show that epidural injections of radio-opaque solutions are not affected by gravity, and that the solutions tend to be distributed rostrally rather more readily than caudally.

Motor blockade

For postoperative analgesia, muscle paralysis is usually unwelcome. There are exceptions — relaxation of muscle spasm related to convulsions of visceral pain or following plastic and reconstructive surgery when immobility may be difficult to maintain voluntarily — but generally loss of function restricts movement, reduces ventilatory capacity, increases the risk to the paralysed part, and increases the difficulties of nursing.

The amount of motor paralysis is dependent upon the identity of the local anaesthetic agent and the time of exposure of the nerve to that agent. Etidocaine and tetracaine produce relatively more motor blockade than bupivacaine and lignocaine; indeed they may block motor nerves in the absence of, or following reversal of, sensory nerve blockade (Table 10.1)

The mechanism for the differences in differential nerve block is uncertain: differences in myelin–lipid solubility are proposed but etidocaine and bupivacaine are highly lipid-soluble, but are very different in this respect; differential penetration of the spinal cord is unlikely, since variable differential nerve block occurs in the peripheral nerves, and the differences in frequency-dependent conduction block are uncertain, since even the large motor fibres have nodes of Ranvier separated by little over 1 mm, and myelinated autonomic fibres are usually more affected than unmyelinated C fibres.

The proportion of motor nerve blockade is increased by increased time of exposure of the nerve to the agents, by the use of vasoconstrictor agents such as adrenaline, or by the use of top-up injections or epidural infusions.

Intercostal nerve blockade

The intercostal space lies below each rib and is formed by the concave surface of the rib above, by the fascia of the internal intercostal muscle laterally, and by the fascia of the intercostales intimi muscles medially. These latter muscles are not attached necessarily to adjacent ribs so the intercostal spaces interconnect (Fig. 10.3). Posteromedial to the angle of the ribs, the internal intercostal and the intercostales intimi muscles are deficient, so that the vein, artery, and nerve (from above down) lie between the internal intercostal fascia and the pleura. The nerve itself usually lies at the level of the lower border of the ribs, but there is considerable anatomical variation (Nunn & Slavin 1980).

Technique

It is recommended that intercostal nerve block is performed just anterior to the angle of the ribs because:
The posteromedial part of the rib moves less than the lateral part, and if the lung is entered it will be torn less at this site.
The rib is identified more easily at the angle than at sites more medial.
Medial to this, the nerve lies on the pleura and lung puncture is more probable.
At the angle, both the lateral and the anterior collateral branches are blocked.

The appropriate ribs should be marked with a skin pen so that intercostal spaces are not injected twice. Following skin sterilization, the skin overlying the rib is retracted rostrally by about ½ cm. A needle is inserted at right angles to the skin to impinge on the rib near its lower edge. The needle is withdrawn and reinserted at right angles but with less skin tension so that it strikes the ribs

Figure showing cross-section of intercostal anatomy with labels: Intercostales intimi, Internal intercostal muscle, External intercostal muscle, Rib, Vein, Artery, Nerve.

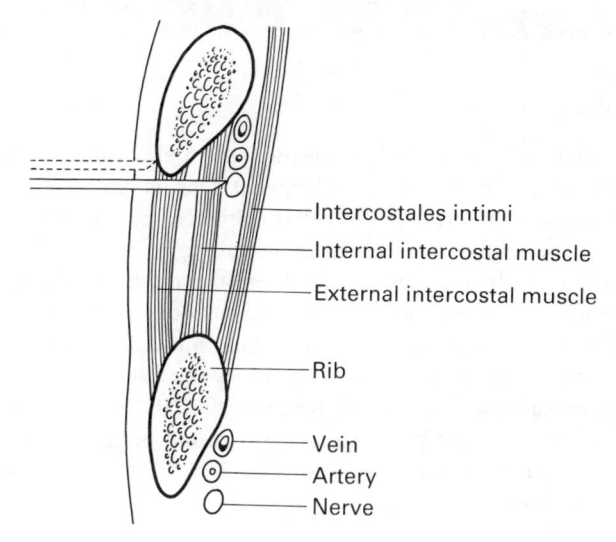

Fig. 10.2.

more caudally. When the lower edge of the rib is reached, if the bevel of the needle is pointed upwards, the needle will glide over the lower edge of the rib. It is inserted a further 3–5 mm or until the needle is felt to pass through the internal intercostal muscle. Aspiration should confirm that the needle tip does not lie in a blood vessel or the lung, and injection of local anaesthetic solution can be made.

For intercostal catheterization, a Tuohy or Crawford needle is used, the needle is directed posteriorly, and the cannula should pass up the subcostal groove. However, the boundaries of the groove are not well defined, and passage of the cannula may be difficult after a centimetre or so.

If a large volume of fluid is used, say 20 ml, more than one space will be filled, and blockade of as many as seven intercostal nerves has been reported from a single injection.

Complications of this technique are, principally, pneumothorax, haemorrhage, and systemic toxicity.

Bilateral subcostal (T12) nerve blocks are very suitable for Pfannenstiel incisions since pneumothorax is very improbable, even if performed during deep inspiration or during intermittent positive-pressure ventilation.

Illiac crest block

Anatomy

The ilioinguinal and iliohypogastric nerves pass through the substance of the psoas muscle and leave it near its lateral edge. They pass around the brim of the pelvis to pierce separately the transversus abdominis muscle. Both nerves, again separately, pierce the internal oblique muscle. However, at, or close to, the anterior superior iliac spine, both nerves and the subcostal nerve lie between the internal and external oblique muscles. Nerve block at this site should provide anaesthesia to the skin anterior to the anterior superior iliac spine, including that above the pubic symphysis, the anterior part of the scrotum and penis, and over the medial part of the groin. It relaxes the lower fibres of the internal oblique muscle.

Technique

Standing on the opposite side of the patient from the nerve to be blocked, the operator places a finger on the lateral (external) aspect of the iliac crest one finger-breadth inferior to its upper margin and three finger-breadths posterior to the anterior spine. The thumb depresses the skin anterior to the anterior superior iliac spine. A short-bevelled needle, at least 2 inches long, is introduced through the skin and directed towards the operator's finger. When it strikes the internal surface of the ilium, it is withdrawn slightly until a relative loss of resistance is detected as the bevel lies in the neurovascular plane between the internal oblique and the transversus abdominis muscles; 10 ml of solution is recommended.

Application. This block is suitable for the pain following herniorrhaphy and bilaterally is usually sufficient for Pfannenstiel incisions (*but see above*). Large-volume injections may block the lateral cutaneous nerve of the thigh, causing numbness and heaviness of the thigh, although muscular power is unaffected.

Caudal blocks in children

In children, the thecal sac may well occupy the majority of the sacral epidural space. The caudal hiatus is to be found superior to the tip of the coccyx by a distance equivalent to two of the patient's phalanges. When the child's hips are flexed to 90°, it is also found to lie in the long axis of the femur. Once the needle has penetrated the sacrococcygeal ligament, it should not be directed rostrally, for fear of penetrating the theca or blood vessels. The following recipe was devised by Armitage (1979):
Bupivacaine 0.25% without adrenaline:

For sacral blocks, e.g. circumcision	0.5 ml/kg
For lumbar and lower thoracic nerves, e.g. herniorrhaphy	1.0 ml/kg
For mid-thoracic nerves, e.g. umbilical hernia repair	1.25 ml/kg

Penile blocks

Penile blocks are effective for operative and postoperative pain in both adults and children. The rate of success is high, and patient discomfort during the block is low.

Injection is made in the midline just below the symphysis pubis (Fig. 10.3). The lower border of the symphysis is palpated with two fingers of one hand. A 25 gauge needle is inserted through the skin, to pass between the fingers, almost to the bone. It is then redirected to pass inferiorly, but not deep, to the symphysis. Following negative aspiration, injection is made.

Recipe. Bupivacaine *without* adrenaline is used:

0–1 years	1 ml
1–5 years	3 ml
6–12 years	4 ml
Over 12 years	5–7 ml

These blocks have been repeated in children in the postoperative period without much discomfort (Muir 1985).

Anaesthesia for the skin

Following split-skin grafts, the donor site may be more painful than the major injury. Application of sterile 1% lignocaine gel or

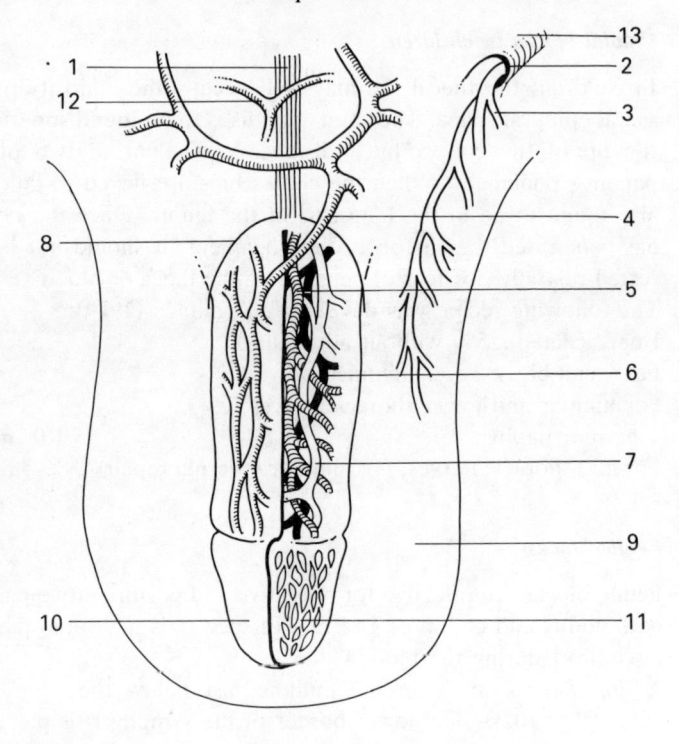

1 Suspensory ligament of penis
2 Subcutaneous inguinal ring
3 Ilioinguinal nerve
4 Superficial dorsal vein of penis
5 Deep dorsal vein of penis
6 Dorsal artery of penis
7 Dorsal nerve of penis
8 Subpubic arch
9 Scrotum
10 Glans penis
11 Plexus cavernosus
12 Anterior cutaneous branch of subcostal nerve
13 Abdominal aponeurosis

Fig. 10.3

ointment to the donor area prior to the dressing with paraffin gauze effectively relieves pain without toxic levels of lignocaine (Bulmer & Duckett 1985). Eutectic mixtures of local anaesthetics (EMLA) applied under an occlusive dressing provide effective anaesthesia to the intact skin. Anti-inflammatory creams, such as benzydamine, provide pain relief when the skin overlying an infusion of irritant substances becomes inflamed.

Following many forms of surgery of the body shell (mastectomy, herniorrhaphy, very low transverse abdominal incisions), the requirement for opioid analgesia can be reduced or eliminated by infiltration of the skin edges with local anaesthetic solution.

Other methods

Psoas sheath block is similar to lumbar sympathetic trunk block, except that the injection is made into the psoas sheath, some 40–50 ml being used. Anaesthesia of the genitofemoral, ilioinguinal, iliohypogastric, femoral, obturator, and lateral cutaneous nerves of the thigh is obtained. It can reduce the pain of femoral neck fractures but, since the 12th thoracic and the sciatic nerves are unblocked, pain in the uppermost part of the lateral thigh and in the posterior thigh and lower leg will be unaffected.

Technique A skin wheal is raised on the same side as the nerve to be blocked, 5 cm from the midline at the level of the second to the fourth lumbar vertebrae. A 22 G nedle is introduced through the wheal at right angles to the skin until the transverse process is encountered approximately 4 cm below the skin. The needle is directed cephalad so that the needle passes over and deep to the transverse process. The injection is made slowly to avoid disruption of the muscle.

Injection made at the medial part of the transverse process will deposit solution between the origins of the psoas muscle and into the paravertebral space. This causes somatic and sympathetic block. Injection deep to the psoas muscle blocks the sympathetic chain.

Paravertebral nerve block produces somatic and visceral pain relief on one side only. In the thorax, it is less likely than intercostal nerve block to produce a pneumothorax. However, it usually requires multiple punctures and carries the risk of dural puncture through a dural cuff or through an intervertebral foramen. It could be used when local anaesthesia is preferable yet when the coagulation status precludes the use of spinal anaesthesia.

Following surgery on, or manipulation of, the knee, complete analgesia can be obtained by *femoral–obturator nerve block*. A short bevelled needle is inserted through the femoral neurovascular sheath just below the inguinal ligament and 1 cm lateral to the femoral artery. Compression of the thigh below the site of injection of 20 ml of local anaesthetic solution causes proximal spread and block of both nerves.

Reversible neurolysis

Neurolysis can be achieved by protoplasmic poisons (e.g. phenol), radiofrequency thermocoagulation, or cryothermy. *Cryothermy* causes degeneration of the axon and myelin sheath, but with preservation of the intraneural and perineural collagen, so that the structure of the nerve pathway is preserved and regeneration is followed by normal function. In contrast to the other methods, inflammation is minimal. Disruption of the axon is caused both by crystal formation during freezing to 60° and by the expansion of the ice and fluid during thawing. Two freeze–thaw cycles are much more effective than one, but the third has less effect. Both sensory and motor nerves are affected, and the technique is probably best reserved for those nerves which are primarily sensory of where motor paralysis is insignificant. In practice, cryoanalgesia is used following thoracotomy and inguinal herniorrhaphy. The nerve can be frozen percutaneously or, preferably, under direct vision at the time of the operation. For effective thoracic analgesia, at least two intercostal nerves on either side of the incision or chest drain must be frozen. Since each freeze–thaw cycle takes between one and two minutes, the technique is time-consuming, and if bilateral analgesia is required it causes considerable intercostal muscle paralysis. The effect lasts for between 10 and 50 days, although prolonged anaesthesia for more than 200 days has been recorded.

Summary

Despite the many possible complications, local anaesthetic techniques can be used for the majority of operations and for the pain in the postoperative period. Indeed, the benefits of local anaesthesia can be greater postoperatively, because the required spread of anaesthesia is usually less and the advantages of being able to move or cough without pain are greater. Some techniques are especially suitable for use in the postoperative period, either by repeated administration or by prolongation of the operative nerve blockade.

CHAPTER 11
Spinally Applied Opioids

Opioids act within the brain and spinal cord to inhibit the perception and emotional effect of noxious stimuli. When exogenous or endogenous opioids are applied to the substantia gelatinosa of the spinal cord, there is inhibition of the slow, dull, burning or aching pain which is associated with the polymodal nociceptors, the spinoreticular pathway, the central parts of the thalamus and diffuse cerebral projections. In higher concentrations, certain opioids, such as morphine or met-enkephalin, reduce the perception of sharper pain. Although the application of opioid to, or stimulation of opioid production at, the dorsal horn of the spinal cord is not as effective as the combined opioid release at the spinal cord and the brain (as shown by studies which cool and depress the descending inhibitory pathways of the cord — *see* Chapter 5), high concentrations of opioids can be applied to the cord without the effects of dangerous central depression, e.g. respiratory depression, stupor, postural hypotension.

Opioids may be applied to the dorsal horn of the cord by iontophoresis (rarely used clinically) or by injection into the cerebrospinal fluid or into the epidural space. Opioids in the subarachnoid space pass principally into the cord, and thence into the systemic venous drainage. A very small proportion diffuses through the dura and epidural capillaries into the systemic circulation. The greater proportion of opioids injected into the epidural space is absorbed into the five litres (approximately) of blood which flows through the epidural circulation, rather than into the relatively static 50 ml of fluid in the subarachnoid space. Nevertheless, the concentration within the cord following either administration will be hundreds or thousands times higher than that which could be achieved by these doses given systemically.

Lipid-soluble opioids are taken up into the cord more quickly and completely from the CSF. They are also washed out more quickly by diffusion into the capillaries of the spinal cord. Water-soluble opioids like morphine are distributed more in the CSF and less in the cord. There exists, therefore, a depot of drug in the CSF, replacing that part of the drug which is eluted from the cord into the systemic circulation. The action of these opioids tends to be longer than that of the more lipid-soluble ones.

The same considerations apply to drugs in the epidural space except that most of the drug is absorbed into the systemic circulation. Even so, epidural opioids have a predominantly regional effect, producing more profound analgesia with lower doses than is possible with systemic administration. The systemic uptake has the additional advantage that the descending inhibitory pathways are activated and that analgesia is provided for the more minor discomforts outside the area of regional analgesia. Although intrathecal administration of opioids can achieve prolonged analgesia — 14 hours with buprenorphine and 48 hours with morphine have been achieved — this is usually inadequate for the whole of the postoperative period, and epidural cannulation with repeated or continuous administration has proved more appropriate.

Cephalad spread of drugs within the CSF is both inevitable and variable. There is no true circulation of fluid within the spinal canal (both descending and ascending flows have been demonstrated, but diffusion and mass movement of CSF cause drugs and radio-opaque chemicals which are injected into the lumbar space to be found in the cerebral cisternae. Radio-opaque chemicals have been shown to move from the lumbar space to the cisternae at the base of the brain 3–6 hours after injection and to remain there for 24 hours. It is assumed that opioids behave similarly and, since the 'respiratory neurones' lie close to the surface of the medulla, late or unexpected respiratory depression may occur even from lumbar injection. This is more likely when water-soluble opioids, which are distributed to the CSF rather than the cord, are used.

The rate and extent of the spread are variable. A strongly regional effect after six hours was noted by Asari *et al.* (1981) for epidural morphine and by Samii *et al.* (1979) for intrathecal morphine. Conversely, Bromage *et al.* (1980) showed that, despite an initial regional effect, segmental hypoalgesia spread centrally after two hours to involve the cervical and cranial segments. Upper thoracic hypoalgesia has been found following lumbar epidural fentanyl, which is very lipid-soluble, albeit following a large bolus injection. This cephalad spread is used by those who inject opioids into the caudal or lumbar epidural space well below the termination of the spinal cord.

The cephalad spread is influenced by the position of the patient, the lipid solubility of the injected opioid, and the rate and volume of administration. Mention has already been made of the disparity of findings with regard to the amount of cephalad spread of the epidural opioid. Despite the 'stirring' effect of movement of the CSF, Gustafsson *et al*. (1982) showed that there was a relative lack of cephalad spread of spinal morphine, as measured by intrathecal morphine concentrations, in those who were mobilized compared to those who were nursed in the horizontal position.

The effect of lipid solubility can be considered by a comparison of morphine and diamorphine. Diamorphine breaks down spontaneously but, in the relative absence of cells, acidity, or sodium ions slowly, to monoacetylmorphine. In cells such as nerve cells, but especially in red blood cells or hepatocytes, it is hydrolysed to morphine. Both diamorphine and monoacetylmorphine are much more lipid-soluble than morphine. The dura mater is a dense fibrous sheet and the transfer of drug across it is influenced by the size of the drug molecule rather than by its lipid solubility. Morphine and diamorphine have similar molecular weights and have almost the same rate of transfer across the dura *in vitro*. However the lipophilic properties affect the amount reaching the CSF because of the differing amounts taken up by the epidural circulation and the epidural fat. The drug can be taken up by the capillaries either through the pores (40 Å in size) or by dissolution in the lipoprotein membrane. The lipid-soluble drugs are absorbed more easily into the systemic circulation and absorbed more easily by the epidural fat.

This latter factor is a theoretical consideration in repeated administration, since the epidural fat could conceivably tend towards saturation, and, similarly, the epidural fat could act as a depot of the drug; neither consideration appears significant in practice.

Thus, the proportion of diamorphine that reaches the CSF is only half that of morphine (Watson *et al*. 1984), although it is twice as effective and diamorphine and morphine are equipotent epidurally. Furthermore, the lipid-soluble diamorphine (or monoacetylmorphine) is cleared from the CSF more than twice as quickly as morphine, and the initial volume of distribution is one-third the size (Moore *et al*. 1984). In summary, the difference in potency of the epidural administration compared to the systemic administration of a lipid-soluble opioid is less than that for a lipid-insoluble one. The lipid-soluble one has a shorter duration because it is cleared more quickly from the spinal cord, but it has a more localized effect and therefore a greater safety because it is distributed more to the cord and less to the mobile phase of the CSF.

As the volume of the epidural injection is increased, so is the cephalad spread of the initial injectate and the chance of cerebral involvement. Equally, the faster the injection is made, the further that injected drug will travel. Just as the absorption of an intrathecally injected drug by a segment of the cord depends upon the speed of the injectate passing across the surface, so the absorption by the cord of an epidurally injected bolus depends on the mass of the drug transferred into the CSF in unit time and the flow of CSF up the cord. Chrubasik *et al.* (1984) have shown that when 2 mg of morphine is injected epidurally in 10 ml of saline, the concentration of morphine in the fourth ventricle is more than 250 times that when the 2 mg is injected epidurally in 1 ml of saline.

Side-effects

Respiratory depression, or, more correctly, ventilatory depression, is the most serious of the side-effects of this technique. It is a consequence of opioid administration by any route and is not uncommon following systemic administration. Minor degrees of ventilatory depression may even improve the efficiency of oxygen uptake by slowing and deepening the ventilation in patients with thoracic or abdominal pain. The dangerous features of the depression in this situation are that it may be severe, sudden, prolonged, and occur after many hours of normal ventilation.

Although ventilatory depression can occur at any time after a bolus injection, a biphasic depression of the ventilatory response to carbon dioxide has been demonstrated, and it is more prevalent at 30 minutes and six hours after epidural administration. It has been suggested that the early depression is due to systemic absorption (Dodson 1985), but severe depression by 2 mg of morphine would be difficult to explain. The later depression is almost certainly caused by cephalad spread within the CSF. *Several opioids* have been implicated. Although it is most common following morphine, ventilatory depression has been reported following alfentanil, diamorphine, fentanyl, methadone, and pethidine, and periods of abnormally slow breathing have been reported following buprenorphine and meptazinol. Two cases of ventilatory depression have been reported when epidural diamorphine was administered in the presence of a dural leak. Almost certainly, these were due to cephalad spread within the CSF, but the depression occurred at 80 minutes and at 4.5 hours (Clarke & Wheatley 1985). If the cephalad flow is *variable*, so is the *concentration* in the CSF. Gustafsson *et al.* (1982) found a 50-fold variation in CSF morphine levels after the same epidural dose. Although the prevalence of ventilatory depression is higher as the dose is increased and if the drug is given intrathecally, depression has occurred after 2 mg of morphine epidurally, and has failed to occur after 16 mg in 45 ml saline given over five hours in a patient who developed heart block and loss of consciousness (Christensen & Brandt 1982).

Age appears to be a factor. Eighteen of the 23 patients with ventilatory depression in the Swedish survey were over 60 years old, and the two above-mentioned patients whose ventilation was depressed following diamorphine were 79 and 84 years old.

Another common factor is the *concomitant use of systemic opioids*. It seems inappropriate that systemic opioids should be required when the central action of the regional opioid is sufficient to depress the ventilation. It is possible that the return of pain reflects a cephalad spread of the drug away from the site of required regional analgesia, and the onset of action of the systemic opioid may coincide with the arrival of the spinal drug at the medulla.

In a survey of 14 000 patients in Sweden (Rawal *et al.* 1987) the prevalence of delayed respiratory depression was estimated to be less than 0.14%. In Brownridge's (1983) study of 9000 boluses of 50 mg of pethidine, given epidurally, naloxone was not indicated or 'contemplated'. The prevalence of ventilatory depression should be compared to that of systemic opioids. When equianalgesic doses of epidural and intramuscular morphine are compared, ventilation and gas exchange are less impaired in those patients given the epidural morphine.

Personal experience. For more than six years, epidural infusions of opioids have been used routinely for thoracic and upper abdominal operations, and many hundreds of patients treated in this way have been nursed on the general postoperative ward. The respiratory rate and pattern are monitored frequently for the first two hours, hourly for 24 hours and two-hourly thereafter until well after the infusion has been discontinued. In almost every case of developing ventilatory depression, it was heralded by slowing of the ventilatory rate and prevented by stopping the infusion. In two elderly patients, naloxone was given to increase the rate. In three patients, the pattern of ventilation became periodic, the response to question became slow, and in one itching developed concurrently. All three symptoms were reversed by naloxone. It may be that this represents a supramedullary spread of opioid and, if untreated, might cause sudden respiratory arrest. In each case, the change in respiratory pattern occurred in the first postoperative hour.

Other side-effects

Pruritis is said by some (Reiz & Westburg 1980) to be segmental, and by others (Bromage *et al.* 1982) to be not segmental and to involve the face. The prevalence is not reduced reliably by the use of preservative-free opioid solutions, and it has been reported after the use of epidural morphine, diamorphine, pethidine, fentanyl, and alfentanil. It may be due to the involvement of the medullary itch centre and thereby represent cephalad spread. It is relieved more by naloxone than by antihistamines.

The reported prevalence of *nausea and vomiting* is very variable. In our own series, it is lower than after systemic opioids. It is especially high following epidural meptazinol and, possibly, after Caesarian section.

Urinary retention is more common in men than in women, and more pronounced in the supine position. It occurs with similar prevalence after intramuscular morphine. Morphine is known to decrease the tone of the detrusor muscle and increase the tone of the internal sphincter. The site of action is uncertain, but the retention is reversed by naloxone. It is more common after morphine, diamorphine and methadone.

Sedation is more prominent after epidural pethidine, buprenorphine, pentazocine and, possibly, alfentanil. Severe sedation may cause respiratory arrest if the airway becomes occluded.

Catatonia has been reported after repeated epidural morphine (Engquist *et al.* 1981). This may be related to the catatonia which is produced by beta-endorphin when injected into the lateral ventricles, and if so is again related to cephalad spread.

Miosis and heart block have also been reported.

Treatment of side-effects is accomplished readily by administration of naloxone, except when buprenorphine or lofentanil has been used, since their receptor binding is such that they cannot be displaced by naloxone. The action of subarachnoid and epidural opioids is prolonged, and the systemic administration of naloxone may be required repeatedly. However, it is capable, when given systemically, of reversing the respiratory depression and other side-effects without necessarily reversing the regional analgesia. Some authors have suggested that intravenous naloxone infusions should be used routinely after spinal opioids where intensive monitoring is not available with certainty.

Choice of drug and technique

Dose and duration

The drug with the longest duration of action is morphine, but the presence of the major part of the drug in the CSF reduces the safety of the technique. A greater proportion of a fat-soluble drug is distributed to the cord, but the rate of loss from the cord into the systemic circulation is also high, such that similar sizes of dose must be used systemically and epidurally, and the epidural toxicity approaches that of systemic administration. Epidural pethidine gives analgesia which lasts between three and five hours, fentanyl gives 2−4 hours of analgesia, but morphine may last for 24 hours or longer. The effect of pethidine can be significantly prolonged by the addition of adrenaline.

Drugs with potent receptor binding have a greater intrinsic duration of effect. Buprenorphine and lofentanil have a relatively long action by any route, and the receptor binding of both is too strong for the action to be be reliably reversed by naloxone; side-effects are therefore less controllable. Buprenorphine has a relatively large molecule; dural transfer is slow compared with systemic uptake from the epidural space so that the ratio of epidural: systemic potency is low.

The *time of onset* of the drug action is also related to the lipid solubility. The concensus of report is that the onset of analgesia after epidural morphine is at 15 minutes and peak analgesia occurs between 30 and 60 minutes after injection. This is very similar to the times of onset following intramuscular administration, and, indeed, following intrathecal administration. This suggests that the delay lies not in the dural transfer but in traversing the lipid membrane and lipid material of the spinal cord (or brain). It is not surprising then that the lipid-soluble opioids have a shorter latency of onset (Bromage *et al*. 1980). The use of added adrenaline does not increase the rapidity of action.

Pentazocine and bremazocine are analgesic by being kappa agonists and possibly therefore mimicking the action of dynorphin (which is found in high concentration in the spinal cord). However, those kappa agonists so far available would not appear to be capable of relieving pains of as wide a variation or of such severity as mu agonists such as morphine.

Diamorphine may be ideally suited to spinal use. It is lipid-soluble and is distributed to the cord rather than to the CSF. Although it traverses the dura less well than morphine, it is equipotent epidurally with morphine. Having entered the spinal cord, it is converted, via monoacetylmorphine, to morphine and has greater difficulty leaving than entering the cord.

The wide variation of *doses* used for regional analgesia reflects the variation of pain experience, the variation of dural transfer, variation of spread within the epidural space and in conjunction with the CSF, and variations of drainage from the spinal cord, metabolism and excretion. Morphine has been studied more than any other drug: 2 mg epidurally proves effective in most cases, but 4 mg is more effective without a signficant concomitant increase in side-effects; 10 mg has been shown to be no more effective analgesically than 5 mg. The prevalence of most side-effects is dose-related, but the range of requirement is so great that there has not been found a single-dose regimen which is effective for all those with thoracic or upper abdominal pain and which does not cause respiratory depression in some patients. In general, the epidural dose is approximately half that of the systemic dose, except for the very lipid-soluble opioids, when doses similar to those used systemically are required. The representative range of doses which have been shown to be effective for acute regional epidural analgesia are:

Morphine	2–7.5 mg
Diamorphine	2–5 mg
Pethidine	25–100 mg
Fentanyl	35–200 µg
Buprenorphine	150–300 µg
Methadone	1–6 mg

Pentazocine, alfentanil, and lofentanil have so far been used by too few workers to be able to determine a representative range.

The intrathecal doses are, on average, about one-tenth to one-quarter those used for epidural analgesia.

Intrathecal or epidural opioids?

Only morphine has been widely used in the subarachnoid space. Intrathecal doses are lower, but, considering that the CSF levels of morphine after intrathecal administration are about 80 times that after the same dose given epidurally, not proportionately so. Since the systemic blood levels after intrathecal administration are very low, it may be that the portion of the epidural dose which is absorbed systemically and distributed to the brain contributes significantly to the analgesia. However, the analgesia is denser, more reliable, and associated with more side-effects (vomiting, pruritis) after intrathecal morphine. *Intrathecal morphine is more effective than epidural morphine for the pain of labour.* High doses of morphine applied directly to a nerve have been shown experimentally to cause loss of sensations other than pain.

Buprenorphine and lofentanil have been used intrathecally. Both are more potent given by this method; the equianalgesic dose of buprenorphine is less than one-fifth that of the epidural one and the duration is more than twice as long. Intrathecal lofentanil is likewise more potent and has a longer duration of action.

Epidural administration remains much more popular. Infusions are more controllable and cannulation allows repeated dosage throughout the period of postoperative pain.

The site of epidural puncture should reflect the site of action of the opioids, which is in the dorsal horn of the spinal cord. The appropriate levels of the cord are those serving the afferent nerves of the wound and are, in the thoracic region, one or two segments higher than those of the vertebral bodies of the spine. The semirecumbent posture encourages the infusion/bolus to travel in a caudal direction, and this opposes the cephalad spread of the drug in the CSF. In practice, injection or infusion at the vertebral level of the upper end of the wound gives effective regional analgesia.

Method of administration. The central effects are less, and the CSF levels in the cisterna magna and the cerebral ventricles are less, when the dose of opioid is given in a low volume, and less still when the dose is given as a slow infusion rather than as a bolus. An infusion has the added advantage that it can be discontinued should untoward effects occur.

The place of spinal opioids in postoperative pain is still controversial. The risk of ventilatory depression exists, even when low-volume intusions of lipid-soluble opioids are used, and continuous monitoring is required. The technique is therefore predominantly used for thoracic and abdominal pain which is difficult to relieve effectively by other means. Nevertheless, those workers, medical and nursing, who use this technique routinely are convinced of its efficacy and relative safety, and many would find ethical objections to returning to alternative methods.

CHAPTER 12
Pain Relief for Problem Patients

Neonates and infants

Problems

1 Do these patients feel pain at all, or, if so, do they feel it in the same way as adults? The trauma and pain of birth are not carried consciously in the memory, and the events of early infancy are similarly not remembered or quickly forgotten. Their influence on later events is doubtful. If the memory and associations of pain are lacking, the affective element is reduced.

Neonates have higher levels of endorphins than adults, and neonatal rats have higher densities of opioid receptors, which decrease during early life. Yet, this does not imply an increased tolerance to pain. A morphine addict also has high levels of opioid but is hyperalgesic during the decline of the hypernormal concentrations. Perhaps the decline in numbers of the opioid receptors prevents or minimizes this supersensitivity to pain.

Neonates and infants cannot communicate their pain and distress verbally, therefore the presence of pain must be inferred by the pattern of behaviour, especially that of crying, expression, and muscular and autonomic responses. Many operations such as squint which cause pain in most adults appear to alter the behaviour pattern very little in most young children and even less in infants. Pain which can be relieved effectively only by opiates in adults appears to be eliminated by the non-narcotic analgesics such as paracetamol.

However, more major operations such as thoracoabdominal procedures and other causes of pain such as haemarthroses and severe glaucoma are associated with changes in the behavioural pattern, and these changes can be reversed by local anaesthesia and opioid analgesia. These changes include:
Alteration of the respiratory pattern, e.g. grunting.
Drawing-up of the knees.

Increase of the heart rate and blood pressure.
Wakefulness.
Change in the facial expression.
Increase of tone and activity of the muscles.
If the pain is severe or prolonged, bradycardia.
Crying.

Crying occurs in response to not only painful stimuli but also hunger, fear, and frustration. It may be possible to distinguish the pattern of cry in response to pain from that due to other factors (Levine & Gordon 1982).

Objective, quantitative evidence is lacking with regard to pain in the neonate and prelingual infant. Certainly, such infants respond to pain such as pin-prick by withdrawal, facial expression, and crying, and it is unlikely that the last two responses are unconscious or spinal reflexes, yet it is possible: a painful stimulus to a comatose patient may cause withdrawal and grimacing, but without memory, distress, or other response. Equally, it is impossible to say that pain is not perceived and found distressing. The grunting, tachycardia, and hypertensive responses found in infants are similar to those found in adults, in whom they are known to be associated with morbidity. It is probable that morbidity and mortality could be reduced by adequate continuous analgesia in these infants.

2 Increased risk of respiratory depression and arrest following opioid analgesics and sedatives. Neonates and infants are more prone to periodic ventilation than adults and sleep a greater proportion of the time. The blood−brain barrier may be deficient, especially in the neonate and the premature infant, and drugs such as morphine pass more easily into the brain. The mechanisms for biotransformation and excretion are more likely to be immature so that the duration of action of drugs is greater. The distribution volume of the drugs is altered, the protein binding may be reduced, and the proportion of extracellular fluid is relatively greater at this age. The sensitivity of the respiratory centre to the opioids is increased (Way *et al.* 1965). Thus, the response of a neonate, especially a premature neonate, to opioids is prolonged and accentuated. In addition to the reduced response of the respiratory centre to carbon dioxide, ventilation may cease without apparent warning of prior respiratory depression. Following opioids, there is depression not only of the bulbar respiratory

'centres', but also of the pontine ones, such that there is a reduction of the respiratory rhythmicity. Those who receive opioids are more reliant on their hypoxic drive. Inhalational agents, e.g. halothane and enflurane, are potent reducers of the hypoxic drive, as are barbiturates, benzodiazepines, and other sedatives and hypnotics. The ventilatory response to carbon dioxide is reduced by sleep and by hyperventilation during the anaesthetic technique, and ventilation may be depressed and more reliant on the hypoxic drive despite normal arterial carbon dioxide levels. It is also probable that the ventilatory response to hypoxia is reduced even in the normal neonate.

3 Although hypersensitivity to the anti-inflammatory group of drugs is unusual in childhood, serum sickness-like reactions may occur in infancy, and an association between aspirin and Reye syndrome has been demonstrated. Reye syndrome is a rare acute encephalopathy associated with fatty change in the liver. It occurs after viral infections, especially those associated with severe pyrexia. The possible association between Reye syndrome and aspirin was sufficient for the United States Food and Drug Administration to warn against using aspirin for influenza and chicken pox. The decline in use of aspirin for children and teenagers (up to 18 years) was followed by a decline in the incidence of Reye syndrome. In the United Kingdom, the age of incidence of Reye syndrome is lower (93% are under 12 years) and the Committee on Safety of Medicines has recommended that children under this age should not be given aspirin unless specifically indicated, say for juvenile rheumatoid arthritis. Paracetamol is equally effective against fever in this age group. The mortality of Reye syndrome is 50%, and many of the survivors are left brain-damaged.

Management of postoperative pain

Most cases of moderate pain can be managed by paracetamol suspension at doses of 60 mg/kg/day. For more severe pain, in infants over the age of one year, morphine 150 µg/kg i.m. or slowly i.v. or pethidine 1 mg/kg i.m. or slowly i.v. can be given. Below the age of one month, opioids should be used with extreme caution and at one-half or one-quarter of this dose unless the patient is already receiving ventilatory support. The newborn infant, and the premature infant who has not achieved his gestational birth age plus one month, are very sensitive to morphine because of the immature blood−brain barrier and because the biotransformation of morphine is likely to be deficient. The effect is likely to be more prolonged than in adults. The use of opioid infusions is gaining in popularity, provided that continuous monitoring of the ventilatory depth and pattern is available. At the very least, this should include apnoea alarms and sufficient nursing staff to be immediately available. Morphine, or papaveretum, pethidine or fentanyl, is commonly used for infusion. Morphine is inefficiently metabolized in neonates and young infants compared to older children, and its active metabolites such as morphine 6-glucuronide may be excreted poorly by the kidney, prolonging the duration of action. The half-life of pethidine is similarly prolonged in the neonate, and the accumulation of pethidinic acid may lead to tachycardia and restlessness. Fentanyl has inactive metabolites and is biotransformed in a number of ways but, nevertheless, the half-life of metabolism may be increased and is predictably prolonged in the presence of raised intra-abdominal pressure (Koehntop *et al.* 1986). However, the distribution of the drug is altered by the different relative volumes of fat and extracellular fluid and reduced circulating blood volume to the extent that it is difficult to judge when the rate of fall of the plasma level of fentanyl changes from that due to redistribution to that due to elimination, and accumulation of effect may occur following a variable period of an apparent steady state. All three drugs have their advocates and are probably as safe and as effective as each other in hands that are experienced in their use. The use of additional sedation increases the risk of respiratory arrest.

The following dose regimen of papaveretum for intravenous infusion is currently in use in Bristol:
Infants, 3 months−1 years   0.02−0.04 mg/kg/hour
Infants under 3 months   0.01−0.02 mg/kg/hour
This compares with a commonly prescribed single intramuscular dose of:
Infants, 3 months−1 year   0.25 mg/kg
Infants under 3 months   0.08 mg/kg

It is suggested that for premature infants under 3 kg, if opioid analgesics are indicated, ventilation should be controlled.

Local anaesthesia, e.g. caudal or penile block after circumcision or repair of the urethra, abdominal wall block for correction of pyloric stenosis, is effective and may eliminate the need for narcotics in some borderline cases.

Obese patients

A patient whose weight is double that of the average for his height may be described as obese.

Problems

These are mainly respiratory: the supine obese patient is hypoxic because of the bulk of flesh pressing on the abdomen and pushing up the diaphragm, compressing the lungs and reducing the surface area for the exchange of gases. Airway closure and gas-trapping is increased. The carbon dioxide tension tends to be increased and the hypoxic drive more prominent. Opioids reduce the hypoxic drive and reduce the drive to ventilate. Airway obstruction, as demonstrated by snoring and periodic breathing, is more common. The muscles are infiltrated by fat and are weaker than their bulk would suggest. Immobility is even more likely to lead to thrombosis and eventual pulmonary embolus. Gastric emptying may be delayed.

Absorption of drugs given by intended intramuscular injection may be delayed because the injection has been into the thick subcutaneous fat. Peripheral veins are more difficult to find and central veins more hazardous to puncture. Local anaesthesia is also more difficult to achieve because of the difficulty of finding the landmarks for injection. It may be contraindicated if heparin has been used for thromboprophylaxis.

The obese patient may suffer from the supine hypotensive syndrome.

Postoperative management

Where possible, the obese patient should be nursed in the sitting or semirecumbent position to ease ventilation and reduce pulmonary compression. The legs should not be dependent unless active, and analgesia should be adequate to enable active mobilization. Drugs should be given intravenously rather than intramuscularly, but continuous intravenous analgesia, or continuous epidural infusion of opioids, local anaesthetics, or both, should be considered. Epidural cannulation may require the use of a 15 cm epidural needle, but these are commercially available and not materially more difficult to use than the conventional needle. Continuous local anaesthetic blockade may be made possible by the insertion of indwelling cannulae at the time of operation. Heparin or other thromboprophylaxis should not be started before insertion of the cannula or before the nerve block.

If analgesia is impossible to achieve without compromising the ventilation, increasing hypercarbia, or inducing hypoxaemia, strong analgesia should be used in combination with controlled ventilation, physiotherapy, and encouragement of active movements.

Postoperative analgesia when raised intracranial pressure is possible

This may be necessary either following intracranial surgery or following surgery to other parts of the body when head injury is present, as when the patient has multiple injuries after a road traffic accident.

Problems

Medication may cause an increase of the intracranial pressure, directly or indirectly, or it may mask the signs of an increasing intracranial pressure. Raised intracranial pressure may show itself by:
Headache, vomiting, and narcosis.
Ptosis and dilation of the pupil which, since it is caused by pressure on the third nerve, may act as a lateralizing sign.
Alteration of the vital signs: increase of the systolic blood pressure and decrease of the diastolic, slowing of the pulse, and irregularities of the ventilation, e.g. hyperpnoea, may be a sign of medullary hypoxia.

Opioid analgesics and local anaesthetics may cause narcosis and slow the pulse. Opioids may cause constriction of the pupil and reduce reactivity. They also tend to reduce ventilation and may, in excess, cause hypercarbia and increase the cerebral blood flow and intracranial pressure; they also reduce the hypoxic drive.

Non-steroidal anti-inflammatory drugs such as aspirin inhibit platelet aggregation and clotting, and may precipitate or increase intracranial bleeding, so that, of the simple analgesics, paracetamol is preferable.

Other analgesics, such as ketamine and nefopam, can raise the blood pressure and the intracranial pressure. Meptazinol causes less ventilatory depression than the other opioids but also reduces the hypoxic drive and is associated with more nausea and vomiting than most; retching and vomiting raise the intracranial pressure.

Management

Fortunately, cranial surgery is not usually followed by severe pain, and paracetamol may suffice. Codeine is frequently used for this condition but it is probable that equianalgesic doses of codeine are no less depressant of the ventilation than morphine. The opioids do not, of themselves, increase the cranial pressure, so that if ventilation is controlled, or if hyperventilation is used to reduce the intracranial pressure, they may be used freely. Similarly, if surgery is necessary, say to repair fractures, anaesthesia with controlled ventilation may be used, but caution should be exercised to ensure that ventilation is normal at the end of the procedure. However, the signs of increasing pressure are disguised and it is often preferable to use local anaesthesia if possible. Here again caution is necessary: large doses of local anaesthetic stimulate the brain and increase its oxygen requirements; inadvertent intravascular injection may cause loss of consciousness and mimic intracerebral haemorrhage, and subarachnoid injection should not be attempted until raised intracerebral pressure has been excluded.

Analgesia for day-case surgery

Patients should be selected for day-case surgery not only on the grounds of ease of or extent of surgery, but also on their fitness for local or general anaesthesia and on their requirement of postoperative analgesia. The medical history, full examination, and desirable laboratory tests should be performed prior to admission, and the results should be available at the time of admission.

Problems

Patients whose medical condition or drug intake reacts adversely with local or general anaesthesia should not be considered. Patients on long-acting insulin, monoamine oxidase inhibitors, or anticoagulants, or with angina, congestive cardiac failure, chronic bronchitis, etc., are in this category. Patients whose postoperative condition demands potent analgesics, e.g. excision of pilonidal sinus or anal fistula, should be admitted even though their condition would not otherwise require specialist nursing.

Patients for day-case surgery should be instructed to abstain from drinking, eating, and smoking for at least six hours before operation, more if they are obese or take antacids, and to abstain from driving or operating machinery for the remainder of the day and night. Yet, it is known that some patients drive themselves home despite the illegality of driving under the influence of drugs, some operate machinery such as cooking stoves, perhaps under pressure from their families, and some undoubtedly drink before operation as shown by the presence of dilute urine in the bladder.

The presence of pain itself is a distraction from activities requiring concentration, but strong analgesics or large amounts of local anaesthetics cause sedation. Both may cause injury.

Management

It is possible to confine day surgical procedures to those following which patients would require only simple analgesics, e.g. cervical dilation, tooth extraction, excision of skin lesions, but most would consider this too exclusive. It is reasonable to use opioid analgesics provided that the peak effect has passed before the patient is discharged home in a fit condition; that further strong analgesia can be confined to that which would produce an effect less than that present on discharge; and further, that the patient is told, and can be trusted, not to drive while under the influence of narcotic drugs.

Local anaesthetic nerve blockade is used widely for day-case surgery and would seem to present little risk in this respect. However, quite large amounts may be used initially and during the procedure, enough to cause material sedation. The patient

Pain Relief for Problem Patients 193

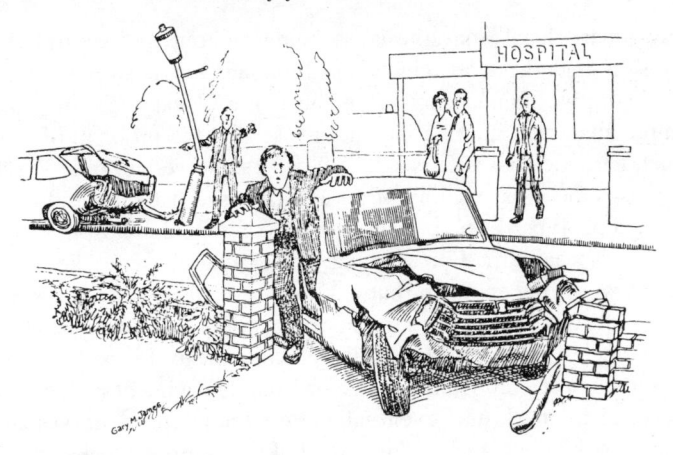

Even local anaesthesia can cause sedation, and patients should not drive or operate machinery.

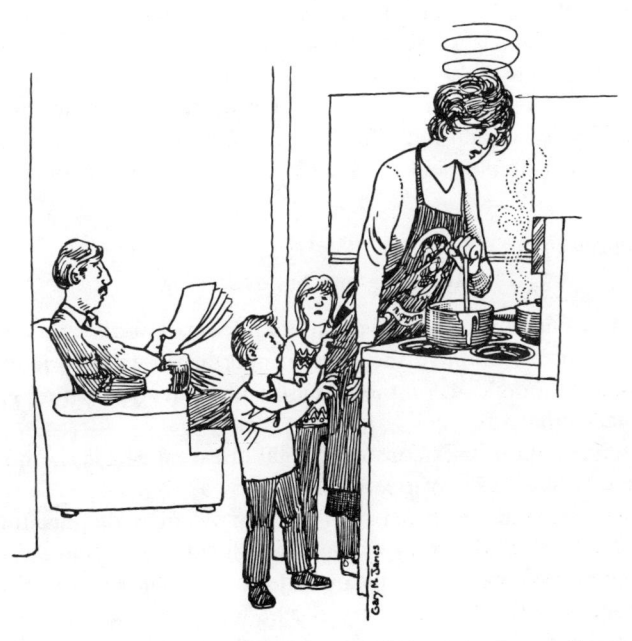

Postoperative day-case surgical patients should not operate machinery: this includes cookers.

may regard local anaesthesia as being without any central depression and drive a vehicle or drink alcohol postoperatively. Postoperative pain occurs when the nerve block wears off, and simple analgesics may be insufficient, so that the problem of how much narcotic analgesia is safe still occurs. Nerve blockade which increases the risk to safety of an unsupervised patient should not be used or, if used, the patient should be retained in hospital until the block wears off. For example, spinal anaesthesia make cause weakness of the legs such that one may give way on the stairs, on the street, etc. This applies to femoral nerve blocks, intra-articular knee blocks, and so on. Following brachial plexus blocks, the arm should be protected from damage or from damaging others. Nerve blocks in the neck may eventually affect the laryngeal nerves and cause choking or the feeling of choking. Nerve blocks which involve the sympathetic system may cause postural hypotension, noticeable only when the patient assumes the upright position suddenly, as when he is called for some form of transport, or if he takes sublingual glyceryl trinitrate for long-standing angina.

Cryoanalgesia provides prolonged analgesia and may be suitable when the field of surgery is served by only one or two sensory nerves. The size of the probe, possible ulceration of the skin or mucosa, and the difficulty of finding a blocked nerve may make it unsuitable, and in many hospitals it is unavailable.

Analgesia and breast feeding

The amount of drug to which the infant is exposed is related to:
1 The concentration of the drug in milk at the time of feeding; this, in turn, depends on the amount and timing of the drug given to the mother.
2 The amount of milk consumed (500–1000 ml per day), and the rate at which it is consumed.
3 The extent to which the drug is absorbed from the intestine.
4 The ability of the baby to metabolize and excrete the drug.

The drug enters the milk by diffusion and the amount that is present depends on:
1 The relative ionization in milk and plasma.
2 The lipid solubility of the unionized form.
3 The relative protein binding in milk and plasma.

Milk is slightly acid relative to plasma, and the highest milk–plasma ratios occur with weakly basic drugs such as the opioids. The rate at which drugs enter the milk depends on the lipid solubility, so that fentanyl exists in the milk soon after administration, and similarly the concentration of fentanyl in the milk falls (albeit slowly) faster than would that of the more water-soluble morphine. Even if the concentration in the milk is low, if the doses are repeated, and the rate of metabolism and excretion in the infant is slow, accumulation will occur.

The newborn or premature infant may not be able to metabolize morphine, and the rate of elimination of other opioids such as pethidine and fentanyl is prolonged. Nevertheless, therapeutic doses of diamorphine, morphine, pethidine, and methadone are unlikely to affect the child (Beeley 1986) and, although repeated use of large amounts by the mother can cause dependence and withdrawal in the infant, it appears to be safe for mothers on methadone maintenance therapy to feed their infants.

Aspirin and aspirin-like drugs are found in the breast milk. The repeated or regular use of large doses of aspirin and other NSAIDs could impair platelet function and produce hypoprothrombinaemia if the vitamin K stores in the neonate are low. Metabolic acidosis in the neonate is possible, and there is a correlation of aspirin use with Reye syndrome in infants and children. Paracetamol would appear to be preferable in lactating mothers, but the amount which can be tolerated by the infant and its immature hepatic metabolism is unknown.

Convulsive pain unrelieved by even high doses of narcotic analgesics

The pain experienced in the central abdomen or in the right side of the abdominal wall following pancreatic and biliary surgery may be due to abdominal wall spasm because of and in addition to biliary or pancreatic duct spasm. Opioids themselves can cause this spasm and make this pain worse. The mechanism can be confirmed by an injection of hyoscine butylbromide 20–40 mg (Buscopan) and can be treated by epidural anaesthesia, intercostal blockade (usually only the right side is necessary), low-dose hyoscine, theophylline, or orphenadrine. Muscle spasm around the large joints following, say, meniscectomy, is due to a sharp pain of movement, poorly relieved by opioids, causing muscle spasm which is not only painful in itself but compresses the joint space and causes further pain. Treatment is by local anaesthesia or by muscle relaxation with drugs such as orphenadrine.

Convulsive pain may be due to abnormal transmission arising from within the nerve itself or because of lack of central inhibition. The most likely cause in the postoperative period is nerve compression, oedema, or damage. Where possible the compression should be relieved; local steroid around the site of compression may relieve the swelling and some of the compression and prevent further damage. Where this is not possible, when irreversible damage has already taken place or when the convulsive pain is long-standing, the pain should be relieved either by local anaesthetics applied as often as is necessary or by anticonvulsive drugs such as carbamazepine, etc. (*see* Chapter 7).

The elderly

Those patients who are elderly often appear unduly sensitive to the actions of analgesics in any form. The response to pain and the demand for analgesia is very variable. Do the elderly require less analgesia and are they less sensitive to pain?

There is little evidence that the elderly (e.g. over 70 years of age) feel less pain, or that the pain causes less change in ventilation or perfusion or behavioural disturbance, than in the case of the young. Experimentally applied pain in the form of pricking or heat applied to the skin may cause less response since the energy absorbed through the aged skin is less. The exaggeration of pain by anxiety may be less, since the elderly probably have fewer dependants, appearance is usually less important, and even the fear of dying may be reduced. It is also possible that those who are easily stressed by external events are less likely to achieve the status of elderly.

It is certainly true that the effects of analgesics and narcotics are greater in the elderly:
1 The volume of distribution of the drug is smaller, especially when the drug is strongly protein-bound. For example, the greater part of morphine in the body is found in the muscle: less muscle — more morphine remaining in the circulation.

2 The processes of biotransformation and excretion are less efficient: as the blood supply to the liver and kidneys decreases, so tha capacity for detoxication and excretion falls. As the oxygenation of these organs falls with age, so does their efficiency.

3 The side-effects of drugs become more pronounced and intolerable. Constipation is more easily caused by the opioids and NSAIDs, urinary retention by the opioids and spinal anaesthesia. Narcosis, i.e. depression of the central nervous system, is greater not only after the opioids, but also after the tranquillizers such as diazepam or phenothiazines. The narcosis is increased by cerebral hypoxia, which occurs gradually as a result of arterial thickening or suddenly as a result of postoperative arterial hypoxaemia. This hypoxaemia may be caused by residual anaesthesia or by abdominal pain (*see* Chapter 4), and since the proportion of pulmonary shunting is greater, the hypoxaemia is less easily relieved by adding oxygen to the inspired gases or air.

4 Epidural anaesthesia is more widespread for a given volume or mass of drug. The ageing of the intervertebral discs causes them to shrink in thickness; the intervertebral foramina become smaller and less local anaesthetic solution is lost through them as the injected solution moves through the spinal canal.

Management

Use a smaller amount of drug until the peak effect of the drug and the effect at steady state can be assessed. Assessment can be relatively rapid if the drug is given initially by the intravenous route. Small amounts at frequent intervals should be able to control the pain, and if the processes of biotransformation and excretion are impaired this interval becomes greater. Epidural anaesthesia requires smaller volume of local anaesthetic, sometimes as little as 40% of the usual volume, but the volume in subarachnoid block is very similar, bearing in mind that the compensatory processes which combat hypotension, such as increase in cardiac stroke volume, are less effective.

CHAPTER 13
Pharmacokinetic Considerations

Pharmacokinetic variability

The amount of pain relief achieved by a given amount of drug depends not only on how the patient is treated by the drug (the amount of pain to be relieved, the efficacy of the drug, the reassuring presence of the administrator), but also on how the drug is treated by the patient. Patients vary in their ability to absorb drugs by the different routes, in the amount of drug which is bound rather than free, in the plasma level of the drug, and in the rate of metabolism and excretion (Fig. 13.1).

Absorption

Drugs may be absorbed into the body by several routes, and the rate of absorption is controlled by the physical properties of the drug and the barrier to absorption. With the exception of the intravenous route (where no barrier exists), the barrier is a cell membrane. Membranes are composed of a double layer of lipid in which are embedded intrinsic proteins such that the ionic groups of the intrinsic proteins are in contact with both the extracellular and intracellular aqueous media. Extrinsic proteins are attached to the surfaces of the intrinsic proteins, but are not involved in the lipid−protein interactions. Drugs may pass across membranes either in aqueous solution through aqueous channels by passive diffusion or by dissolving in the lipoprotein membrane itself. The transfer depends upon the concentration gradient. If the drug is ionized, it depends also upon the difference in electrical charge across the membrane. It depends, therefore, upon the pH of the solution on either side of the membrane, and on the pK of the drug (the pH at which there is 50% ionization).

The size of the membrane channels differs in different sites. Capillary endothelial cells have large channels with a diameter of 40 Å, whereas the channels in the red cell membrane, the

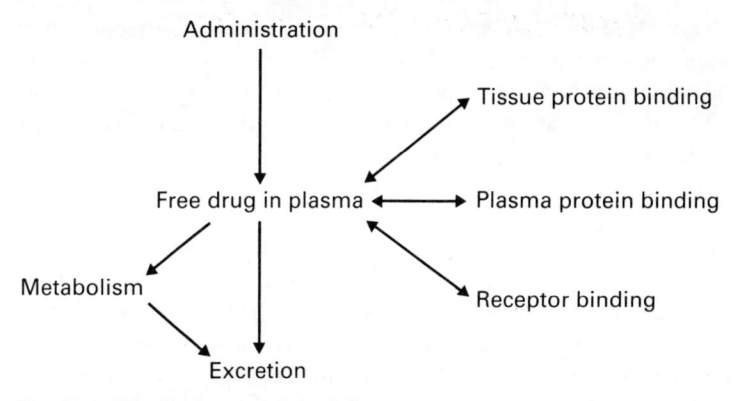

```
                    Administration
                          |
                          |           → Tissue protein binding
                          |          ╱
                          ▼         ╱
          Free drug in plasma ←────→ Plasma protein binding
              ╱       |       ↖
             ╱        |         ↘
     Metabolism       |          Receptor binding
             ↘        ▼
               Excretion
```

Fig. 13.1. Distribution and fate of drugs.

intestinal epithelium, and most cell membranes in the blood–brain barrier have a diameter of 4 Å and allow the transfer only of water and small water-soluble molecules with a molecular weight less than 200.

The rate of absorption is related to the concentration gradient (drugs in high concentration are absorbed more quickly than drugs in low concentration), the perfusion of the absorptive site, (which maintains the gradient), and the surface area available for absorption. Where the regional perfusion is reduced, as in shock or general anaesthesia, absorption may be delayed. Vasoconstrictor substances such as adrenaline are used in conjunction with local anaesthetics deliberately to delay absorption.

Oral administration

This is the most common method, the most convenient, and the most economical. Administration involves little or no discomfort, self-administration is easy, and the drug is not required to be sterile. The gastric and intestinal mucosa can be considered as a continuous lipid layer with small channels of transfer. Absorption therefore is almost entirely in the non-ionized form. Weak acids such as acetylsalicylic acid can be absorbed through the gastric mucosa, and weak bases such as morphine and paracetamol are absorbed almost entirely in the small intestine. The solubility of the drug is also a factor. Aspirin is very insoluble in its unionized form; even soluble aspirin may flocculate in the stomach, and the amount of drug in contact with the absorbing surface is then relatively small. Drugs which are given in the solid form may dissolve slowly and pass by the areas of optimal absorption before dissolution. The same problems occur with enteric-coated capsules or time-release capsules.

Topical application

The skin and mucous membranes also have small pores in the cell membrane; drugs therefore are mainly absorbed in their unionized form. Drugs may be given in this way for their local effects, e.g. local anaesthetics, or for their general effects, e.g. glyceryl trinitrate. Absorption of a drug through the skin will depend on the site, for example the skin of the perineum is more absorptive than that of the dorsum of the hand. Abrasion of the skin, inflammation, and other conditions which enhance cutaneous blood flow also aid absorption. Benzydamine cream increases dermal blood flow, and thereby the penetration of the drug. Rubbing the skin can increase penetration, as can the use of an occlusive dressing which causes maceration of the skin by retaining moisture.

The sublingual and rectal routes of administration

These routes have the additional benefit that the drug does not pass through the liver before entry into the systemic circulation. Rectal absorption is often irregular and incomplete, and some drugs cause irritation of the rectal mucosa. However, rectal routes can be used when oral ingestion is unreliable because of an unknown gastric transit time or during unconsciousness. Sublingual administration is more certain, and the drug is also protected from rapid inactivation by the liver since venous drainage for the mouth is to the superior vena cava. In the presence of salivation much of the drug will be swallowed and in the presence of unconsciousness the tablet may be inhaled.

Intravenous administration

This is the most certain method of all. The concentration within the plasma can be judged with accuracy and can be achieved almost immediately. The dose of the drug can be titrated against the response of the patient, and the drug, if given slowly, is greatly diluted; this route may be the one of choice in the case of irritant substances such as thiopentone. However, oily drugs are not suitable and solubilizing agents such as propylene glycol and cremaphor EL may have disadvantages of their own.

Intramuscular and subcutaneous injection

These routes provide a slower and more constant absorption. However, they are subject to the influence of regional perfusion of the site of injection, and this may render them unsuitable in the case of shock. The pores in the cells of the capillary endothelium are large, and the absorption into the bloodstream depends more upon the perfusion and the solubility of the drug at the pH of tissue and plasma than upon its lipid solubility. Nevertheless, depot preparations can be made by incorporating the drug into an oily substance or as a solid pellet so that absorption is delayed. So far, the simple analgesics have not been used in this way.

Pulmonary absorption

This route is used largely for gaseous and volatile drugs. Ephedrine and other bronchodilators are used in this way, and of course opium has been smoked for many centuries. Again the absorption is variable. They are absorbed through the pulmonary epithelium and mucous membranes in the respiratory tract. The surface area for absorption is very large, but the absorption of any given dose is variable. Drugs may also be nebulized and inhaled.

Bioavailability

Drugs may be chemically equivalent if they contain the same weight of drug in each preparation. Bioavailability is the term used to describe the amount of drug which is available to the body, i.e. the proportion which is absorbed into the bloodstream. Enteric-coated tablets, for example, may be so resistant to absorption that they pass out unchanged and the drug has little bioavailability. Differences in bioavailability result from differences in crystal form and particle size, and refer especially to oral administration. Bioavailability may be delayed if the tablets are given in dry form, as an insoluble compound, or in the recumbent position, because of delay in the oesophagus. The availability of paracetamol varies from 63 to 89%. Many drugs such as the opioids have a high first-pass metabolism, i.e. they are metabolized in the liver and the gut wall and are not able to exert their effects on target organs. The bioavailability of morphine varies from 20 to 100% (McQuay & Moore 1984). Most authorities recognize that it is one-third to one-half as potent when given orally as when given systemically. The bioavailability of oral morphine given regularly for pain during terminal care is assessed at 50% of the intramuscular dose (Saunders 1981).

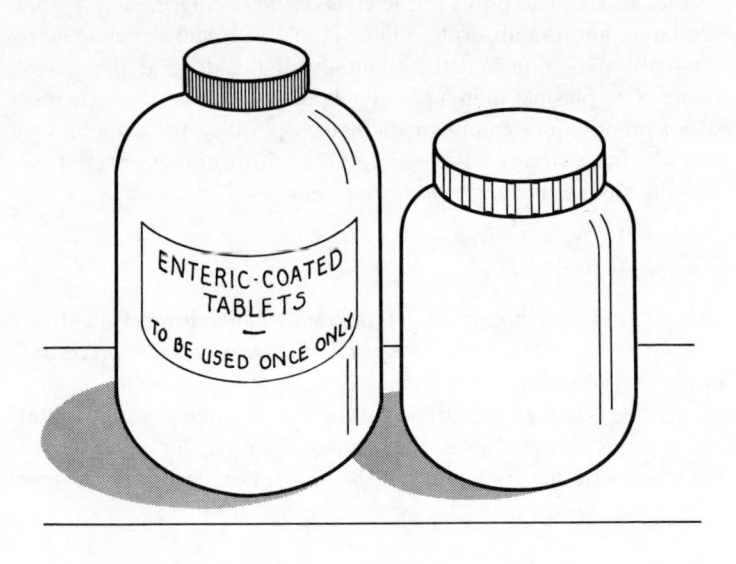

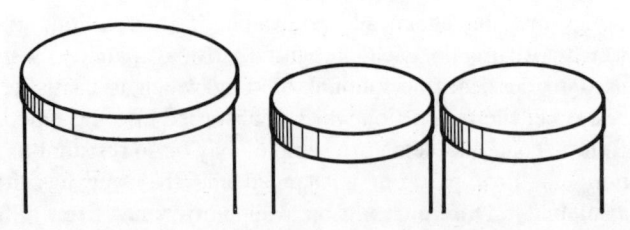

Enteric-coated drugs may have little bioavailability

Distribution

Following administration by any route, the drug is absorbed into the plasma and thence distributed to the tissues of the body. Initially, the greatest amount of drug is distributed to those organs which have the greatest blood flow; the concentration in these organs will approach that of plasma (Figs 13.2 & 13.3). At the same time, tissues with a less rich blood supply will be taking up drugs more slowly. The level in the plasma falls because of the distribution to tissues, and falls to a level below that of the well-perfused tissues. A concentration gradient now exists agains between the well-

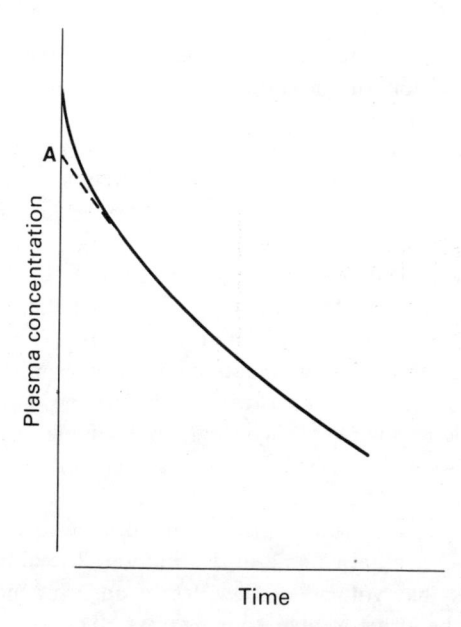

Fig. 13.2. Plasma levels following an intravenous dose of a drug. The solid line demonstrates two curves: an initial one which is due to the redistribution of the drug, and a second flatter one which is due principally to its elimination. The concentration at A is that which would have been obtained if there were instantaneous distribution of the drug throughout the body.

$$\text{The } \textit{volume} \text{ of distribution} = \frac{\text{Dose administered}}{\text{Concentration at A}}$$

perfused tissues and the plasma, and the concentration in the well-perfused tissues falls. The drug is distributed, at equilibrium, throughout the body according to the capacity of the tissues to contain the drug in solution. For example, although the concentration of morphine in skeletal muscle is lower than that in the liver, kidney and spleen, because of the mass of muscle, the greatest proportion of administered morphine exists in muscle; conversely the greatest proportion of a lipid-soluble drug such as fentanyl is found, after redistribution, in the body's fat deposits.

Lipid-soluble and lipid-insoluble are relative terms since most drugs have the ability to dissolve in both fat and water in differing proportions. This is partly governed by the degree of ionization, which depends not only on the dissociation constant of the drug but also on the pH of the body fluid at the site under consideration.

Equilibrium is never reached because, except in rare circumstances, elimination of the drug is occurring almost from the moment of administration.

Drugs may be bound to tissue proteins and plasma proteins and, in the bound form, cannot pass across membranes, act at the drug receptor, and, under most circumstances, be eliminated. The bound portion represents a reservoir of drug which will contribute to the duration rather than intensity of effect.

The volume of distribution is the volume calculated from the dose of the drug administered and the plasma concentration, having made allowance for elimination of the drug. A lipid-soluble drug such as fentanyl passes across the membrane barriers more quickly and more completely than a 'lipid-insoluble' drug such as morphine. A smaller proportion of fentanyl remains in the plasma, and the apparent initial distribution volume is greater. The distribution volume is reduced by surgery and/or anaesthesia (Stanski *et al*. 1978). The initial volume of distribution (V_1) of an intravenous bolus is that volume of the plasma and that part of the tissues that the drug is able to penetrate. The penetration is confined mainly to perfusion-rich tissues such as brain, heart, kidney, liver, spleen. The concentration of drug in these tissues, initially high, falls mainly because of redistribution. The rate of fall of concentration because of redistribution is related to the concentration and the volume of distribution (because of redistribution), and the theoretical time taken for the concentration to fall to 50% is called the redistribution half-life ($T_{1/2}$ or $T_{1/2\alpha}$).

The total volume of distribution at a steady state represents the volume of drug following redistribution. Tissue protein binding increases, and plasma protein binding decreases, the apparent volume, since most assays measure the total drug in the plasma, free and protein-bound, ionized and unionized. The volume of distribution at steady state is the relationship of the concentration of the drug in the plasma to the amount given, calculated when the concentration is maintained at a constant level by infusion or when the infusion rate is constant. Thereby, the further redistribution consequent on drug elimination is reduced or avoided. These volumes can be used to calculate loading doses and infusion rates to achieve and maintain analgesia without under- or overdosage.

The more quickly the drug is administerd, e.g. by intravenous bolus, the higher the initial concentration and the greater the central effect. A slower, e.g. intramuscular, administration would require a larger dose to achieve the same effect, but the effect would last longer because redistribution occurs during administration, depending upon the rate of absorption and the rate of elimination (Fig. 13.3). When a lipid-soluble drug such as fentanyl is given, the decline in effect of a small dose is predominantly due to redistribution; when a large dose is given, such that the capacity of the lipid site to absorb the drug is approached, the decline in effect is predominantly due to elimination. The duration of analgesic or respiratory depressive activity of fentanyl is not linearly related to the size of the dose.

Maintenance of a constant blood level

In any individual, the range of concentration of analgesic drug which is associated with effective analgesia without toxic side-effects is narrow, but may be achieved and maintained by the application of pharmacokinetic principles.

The desired effect can be achieved by titration of the drug against the patient's response. The quickest, most reliable, route for most drugs is intravenous. Thereafter, the fall in plasma level, first by redistribution then by elimination, is corrected by controlled administration. For the initial correction, intravenous infusion is most suitable, but for slow administration other routes such as transdermal, subcutaneous, sublingual, intramuscular or,

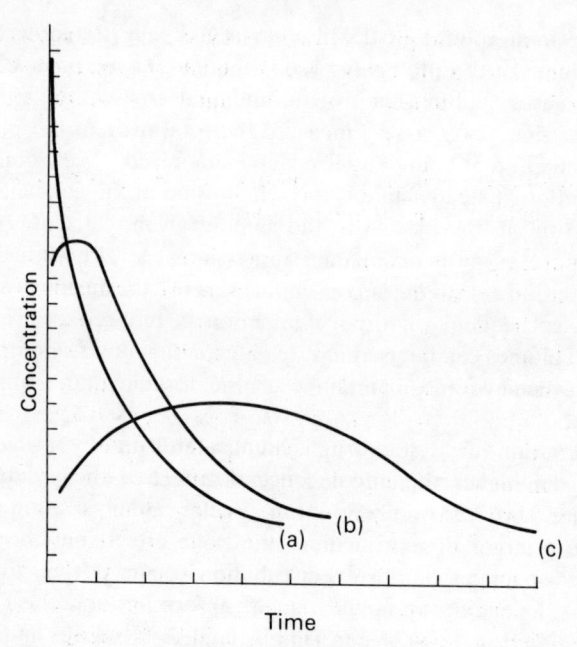

Fig. 13.3. These curves show the concentration of drug following intravenous administration in (a) plasma, (b) tissues with moderately high perfusion, e.g. liver, kidney, and (c) tissues with low perfusion such as muscle and fat. The same curves demonstrate the plasma levels of a drug following (a) intravenous administration, (b) intramuscular administration, (c) subcutaneous or oral administration.

occasionally, oral can be used. The considerations of spinal or regional analgesia are dissimilar and are considered separately (*see* pp. 164 & 175 *et seq.*).

The redistribution of the drug and its elimination are exponential, i.e. the plasma level is reduced to 50% in one unit of time called half-life, and to 25% in another, etc. The concentration in the plasma (C_p) is equal to the fraction of the dose (F) which is absorbed multiplied by the dose frequency (f) divided by the volume of distribution (V_D) and an elimination constant (K_{cl}).

$$C_P = \frac{F \times f}{V_D \times K_{cl}} = F \times f \times \frac{T_{1/2}}{0.69} \times \frac{1}{V_D}$$

If the dose of the drug is given at intervals equal to the half-life of the drug, and given intravenously so that the absorption is complete, the plasma concentration equals the dose of the drug divided by the volume of distribution and 0.69 (natural logarithm of 2).

Mean plasma concentration = dose × 1.44 divided by volume of distribution (as 1.44 is the reciprocal of the natural logarithm of 2)

If the drug is given by intravenous infusion without an initial bolus, the calculated concentration is nearly reached after four half-lives. In the case of morphine or fentanyl this is of the order of 12–16 hours, and too long to be useful. The size and rate of administration of the initial bolus must depend upon the size of the initial volume of distribution and the required level of analgesia. If the bolus which achieves optimum effect is given too rapidly, the level of analgesic falls to ineffective levels before the body has absorbed enough drug from the constant administration, or it must be larger than that required for effective analgesia without toxic effects. The bolus may be given at a decreasing rate to allow for redistribution, or may be given in decreasing increments. Alternatively, it can be given in high dosage at a time when the toxic effects, such as ventilatory depression, nausea, itching, have no significance, such as during balanced anaesthesia, provided that the operation is of sufficient duration to allow the analgesic level to decline to that required. At the same time, a constant infusion is initiated to replace losses from biotransformation and elimination. Although subcutaneous infusions have been used satisfactorily (Goudie *et al.* 1985) postoperatively, the changes in regional blood flow to the skin render them less satisfactory than intravenous infusion. There is conflicting evidence for the development of tolerance during postoperative infusions and the declining analgesic requirement may make clarification difficult.

Biotransformation and elimination

Some analgesic drugs are eliminated through the lungs with little if any change, e.g. nitrous oxide, some are secreted into the milk and gastric contents, e.g. morphine, pethidine, fentanyl, and some are excreted unchanged by the kidney (morphine 6–19%,

Table 13.1. Pharmacokinetic data of some opioids in healthy volunteers or anaesthetized subjects.

Drug	Morphine	Pethidine	Fentanyl	Alfentanil
Intravenous dose (mg)	3.5–14	25–350	0.1–2.2	0.2–18
Redistribution half-life (minutes)	9–20	3.3–17[1]	1.2–25	5.1–19
Elimination half-life (hours)	1.7–4.5	2.4–6.7	1.7–14[2]	1.4–1.6
Initial distribution volume (l/kg)	0.04–0.33	0.6–2.2	0.04–1.27	0.08–0.22
Total distribution volume (l/kg)	1.2–4.7	2.7–5.9	0.7–4.2	0.39–1.0
Clearance (ml kg^{-1} min^{-1})	6.4–23	7.5–23	1.9–22[3]	3.2–8.3
Plasma binding (%)	35	58	84	92

Notes
1 One study yielded an uncharacteristic result of 30 minutes.
2 Depending on dose — *see text*.
3 1.9–6.3 for anaesthetized subjects; 10–22 for awake volunteers.

pethidine 4–22%, indomethacin 10–20%). However, the majority of analgesic drugs are metabolized (biotransformed) before excretion by the kidney. The metabolites are generally less active than the administered drug, although this is not always the case. Diamorphine, phenacetin and sulindac depend for their analgesic effect upon biotransformation to active metabolites. The metabolite of aspirin by hydrolysis—salicylic acid—is active but too irritant to be administered by mouth itself. Some metabolites are responsible for the side-effects of the analgesic drugs: convulsions and confusion by norpethidine; the dizziness of lignocaine toxicity (Boyes *et al.* 1971); the allergic phenomena of the ester-type local anaesthetics (by para-aminobenzoic acid); and the methaemoglobinaemia of prilocaine (*o*-toluidine) and paracetamol. Most metabolites are polar, water-soluble molecules, and are not reabsorbed by the renal tubules and are less able to cross the blood–brain barrier or cross the neural membrane. (The polar morphine 6-

glucuronide is active when injected directly into the CSF or when present in the plasma in high concentrations.)

The biotransformation of drugs may be synthetic or non-synthetic. The non-synthetic transformations involve oxidation, reduction, or hydrolysis: they are sometimes called phase I reactions. The synthetic or phase II reactions involve conjugation, usually with glucuronic acid derived from glucose. The enzymes involved in the biotransformation of most analgesics are located in the smooth endoplasmic reticulum of the liver, although these enzymes are also present, to a lesser degree, in other tissues such as the kidney, gastrointestinal tract, and plasma. This reticulum is also known as the microsomes because of its appearance after centrifugation. The hepatic microsomal enzyme system catalyses glucuronic conjugation and most oxidative drug reactions. The liver has a very large capacity for conjugation, especially with glucuronide, except in the neonate and premature infants. Reduced conjugating capacity leads to hyperbilirubinaemia and increased sensitivity to morphine. The neonate and premature infant also have a poorly developed blood–brain barrier and an immature mechanism for excretion, which increase the sensitivity to opioids. Opioids, especially morphine and its cogeners, should be used with great caution prior to delivery of the infant and during lactation and breast-feeding of the newborn or for surgery of the neonate himself. Glucuronides are secreted into the bile and urine. Bile glucuronides are excreted into the small intestine, where some may be hydrolysed. Glucuronide conjugation is involved in the biotransformation of analgesic drugs such as morphine, naloxone, pentazocine, indomethacin, and paracetamol.

Hepatic microsomal oxidative reactions involve molecular oxygen, reduced nicotinamide adenine dinucleotide phosphate (NADPH), and cytochrome P_{450} and its reductase. The rate of biotransformation is influenced by many competing endogenous and exogenous substrates, including carbon monoxide at concentrations found in heavy smokers. Oxidation is involved in the biotransformation of lignocaine and of pethidine to norpethidine.

The capacity for microsomal oxidation is comparatively limited, and the half-life of pethidine may be increased by up to 100% by viral hepatitis or cirrhosis, whereas the disposition of morphine is unaltered in these conditions. The plasma protein binding is not altered by hepatitis, and the increased half-life of pethidine results from delayed hepatic clearance. Morphine and fentanyl (which is also unaffected) are preferable in these conditions. Non-microsomal drug transformation occurs mainly in the liver but also in the plasma and other tissues. For example, ester-type local anaesthetics are hydrolysed by cholinesterases such as plasma cholinesterase. *Hydrolysis* of glucuronide conjugates may occur in the gastrointestinal tract, thereby releasing active drugs which are once more absorbed into the bloodstream — the enterohepatic circulation. Indeed all conjugation, other than with glucuronide, and some oxidation, reduction, and hydrolysis, occur outside the microsomal system. For example, salicylic acid is conjugated with glycine, and paracetamol is partly conjugated with sulphuric acid (35%).

Excretion

Drugs may be excreted either unchanged or as metabolites. Vapours and gases are excreted by the lungs. Solutions and solids are excreted by the kidneys and the bowel, and to a lesser extent by the sweat, saliva, tears, and milk. Vomit and other forms of loss are pathological but postoperatively may account for an unknown amount of loss of drug. Many metabolites formed in the liver are excreted into the intestine in the bile. Indeed organic ions are secreted actively into the bile and thence into the faeces. However, others like glucuronide are partly hydrolysed in the intestinal tract and the base reabsorbed to be remetabolized and subsequently excreted in the urine. The kidney is therefore the most important organ for elimination of drugs. Excretion involves three processes: glomerular filtration, active tubular secretion, and tubular reabsorption. The amount of drug passing into the glomerular filtrate depends upon the glomerular filtration rate and the amount which is bound to plasma proteins. In the proximal renal tubule other drugs are added to the filtrate by active secretion, e.g. glucuronides. In the proximal distal tubules the unionized forms of drugs and their metabolites are reabsorbed, whereas the ionized forms are are unable to pass across the tubular membrane. Thus any form of biotransformation which converts the drug into an ionized form will promote excretion. Alkalinization of the urine will promote elimination of acids such as salicylic acid.

Pethidine and fentanyl may be found in the gastric juice since these drugs are strongly ionized in the acid submucosa and gastric secretions. Reabsorption is very slow until the drugs pass into the alkaline medium of the small intestine. Similarly, milk, which is more acid than plasma, will concentrate such basic compounds. Non-ionic compounds such as ethanol are concentrated to the same extent in the milk as in plasma.

Time of elimination and clearance of drug

If the processes of biotransformation and elimination have a capacity which exceeds the demand, the rate of elimination of drug will be proportional to the concentration of the drug. The half-life ($T_{1/2}$) of elimination ($T_{1/2\beta}$) will be the time taken for the concentration of the drug to be 50% of that at theoretical immediate distribution. The body will be 50% cleared of the drug in one half-life, 75% clear in two half-lives, 88% in three and 94% in four half-lives. A constant fraction of the drug present is eliminated each unit of time, and this is known as first-order kinetics. With some drugs, the biotransformation–elimination processes are saturated, and the rate of elimination is not proportional to the concentration of the drug; a constant amount of drug present is eliminated per unit of time, and the time for elimination will be determined by the total dose of that drug. This is known as a zero-order kinetics.

Another value often quoted is the volume of blood which is totally cleared of drug in unit time. Thus if the volume of distribution is large, the plasma concentration is low, the concentration gradient across the organ of elimination is small, and the clearance of the drug from the body is slow (*see also under* Renal excretion). The rate constant of the first-order kinetic process and the half-time or half-life ($T_{1/2}$) are simply related ($K_{el} \cdot T_{1/2} = 0.693$), as are the half-life, the volume of distribution and the clearance (Cl).

$$T_{1/2} = \frac{0.69\ V_D}{Cl}$$

Implications

Size of dose

Austin *et al.* (1980) have shown that individual patients are remarkably consistent in the concentration of pethidine required to produce analgesia and that the differences in drug concentration between that of a patient experiencing severe pain and that of the same patient experiencing little or no pain can be very small. However, they also showed that the blood concentration of pethidine giving effective analgesia in *different* patients varied from 0.27 to 0.70 mg/l. There is also considerable variation in the dose required to yield a given plasma concentration. Doses of pethidine (and other drugs) administered directly or indirectly into the plasma should be varied according to the patient and the response. The individual variation when opioids are injected directly into or around the central nervous system is not so well established. There is also considerable pharmacokinetic variation.

Factors affecting the variability of analgesic distribution and elimination

Size of dose

There is no evidence that biotransformation of even very large doses of opioids in normal individuals is changed from first-order to zero-order kinetics, i.e. that the biotransformation processes become saturated. The possibility remains that this may occur where the biotransformation processes are already compromised, for example in the neonate or in the presence of hepatocellular damage. However, some of the effects of the drug may alter its rate of elimination. Hepatic blood flow may decrease acutely after beta-adrenergic blockade or during hypotension caused by sympathetic blockade. Such may occur following regional blockade with lignocaine; hepatic blood flow is reduced, and hepatic clearance of lignocaine, which is high, will also be reduced. The size of dose of those drugs subject to zero-order kinetics, such as salicylic acids, determines the time of elimination.

Age

There is little difference in the pharmacokinetics of the opioids or other analgesics in those infants more than one month old and in adults. Neonates, i.e. infants less than one month old, and especially premature neonates, show an immaturity of the conjugating system of the microsomal enzymes, and the glucuronidation of morphine is impaired. Paracetamol is excreted predominantly as a sulphate, whereas in adults it is predominantly the glucuronide which is eliminated. In neonates the half-life of pethidine is seven times greater than in adults (Caldwell *et al.* 1978), and that of fentanyl is 1.5−3 times that of the average of the general population (Koehntop *et al.* 1986). In both the aged and in neonates the low level of plasma proteins increases the unbound fraction of the drug in plasma. Also, the cardiovascular changes associated with ageing may slow the distribution of the drug to the liver and kidneys and other peripheral tissues so that the decline in morphine levels in plasma is more gradual. Bentley *et al.* (1982) showed that although the terminal elimination half-life of fentanyl is more than doubled in elderly patients as a result in the decrease in drug clearance, the volume of distribution is unchanged. Thus serum fentanyl concentrations, and indeed serum pethidine concentrations, are higher in patients of 70 years or older, for a given dose, than in younger patients. The volume of distribution of pethidine has also been shown to be unchanged by age. In the elderly both impaired metabolism and decrease in hepatic blood flow occur. Hepatic blood flow may be decreased by as much as 45% in older patients resulting from a combination of reduced cardiac output and reduced total liver activity.

Gender

Rigg *et al.* (1978) showed a significant difference in the elimination half-life of morphine between males (mean 173 minutes) and females (mean 110 minutes). This could be explained by the increased muscle mass in males, and the difference may not be as great for more lipid-soluble drugs.

Body weight

In neonates and children the dose is calculated on the body weight, and this is probably valid where the lean body mass is similar. Bentley *et al.* (1982), who studied the disposition of fentanyl in normal and obese patients, concluded that blood concentration was independent of body weight. Furthermore, the half-life and volume of distribution were similar in both obese and normal patients.

In the obese, gastric emptying may be reduced, and the rate of absorption of an orally administered drug may be reduced. Intramuscular injection may be mistakenly assumed when the injectate has been given into a fatty deposit over the intramuscular site. Absorption will therefore be slower than expected.

Preoperative anxiety

Preoperative anxiety leads to vasoconstriction, and may explain the slower absorption of pethidine from intramuscular sites and its reduced volume of distribution in surgical patients. Plasma concentrations of intramuscular pethidine increase suddenly upon the induction of anaesthesia (Mather *et al.* 1975) because of the vasodilating effects of anaesthetic agents.

Anaesthesia and surgery

There are cardiovascular changes consequent on anaesthesia in surgery, and the two factors have not been completely separated. Operated patients redistribute pethidine more quickly than awake control subjects; there is a reduced initial volume of distribution and a tendency for the clearance of steady-state distribution volume to be lower. This is probably due to reduction in tissue perfusion and hepatic and renal blood flow. However, in individual studies the reduction in clearance and distribution volumes is relatively small in general surgical patients compared to volunteers.

Greater pharmacokinetic differences occur with fentanyl in patients undergoing cardiac surgery with extracorporeal circulation. There is considerable haemodilution but, providing the analgesic drugs are given prior to cardiac bypass, most of the drug will be distributed to the tissues. The plasma concentration of the drug, especially that not bound to plasma proteins, will be maintained relative to the degree of increase of volume of distribution, since plasma proteins are increased less than the volume of blood. Hypothermia will reduce the rate of drug biotransformation, and the exclusion of the lungs from the circulation preserves a store of drug which will be available once normal circulation is re-established. After surgery inotropic, chronotropic, and vasoactive drugs would all be expected to alter the disposition of any analgesics administered.

Ventilation and acid-base balance

Opioids. Respiratory acidosis, i.e. retention of carbon dioxide, increases the proportion of drug that is ionized in plasma, decreases the amount of opioid bound to plasma proteins, increases the ionization of the drug in the brain, and increases cerebral blood flow. There is decreased renal tubular reabsorption from the acid glomerular filtrate, but there is a larger distribution volume so that the elimination half-time is unchanged. Because of these opposing effects on the penetration into, and retention by, the central nervous system, the brain levels of morphine are found to be higher in both hypo- and hypercapnia. In hypocapnia in dogs the higher brain:plasma concentration ratio reflects the degree of unionization of the drug in its ability to enter the brain. In hypercapnia the higher brain morphine levels reflect the decreased plasma protein binding, the higher plasma levels of morphine, and the greater cerebral blood flow. In hypercapnia there is also a slower rate of decline of the brain morphine levels because of the greater ionization within the cells of the brain.

The convulsive threshold to local anaesthetics is also related to the arterial tension of carbon dioxide. An increased arterial carbon dioxide tension is associated with a reduction in the blood level of local anaesthetic required to produce convulsions, and a decrease in carbon dioxide tension is associated with an elevation of the blood level required for convulsions. The effects of pH are additive, i.e. high carbon dioxide tension and decreased pH decrease the convulsive threshold more than the same high carbon dioxide tension with a normal or elevated pH. The explanation of this is not certain. Acidosis and the increased ionization of the drug would reduce penetration into the central nervous system; the ionization within this brain cell would tend to increase its activity. The increase in cerebral blood flow may be the most important factor. Acidification of the urine would enhance its excretion, yet this is not an advisable method of treatment for toxic symptoms because of the above considerations. Similarly, any factor which causes local extracellular acidosis at the site of injection will increase ionization of the drug and reduce diffusion of local anaesthetic base into the nerve. Local anaesthetic injections themselves are acidic; the depletion of the buffer capacity at the site of injection, for example within the spinal column, is one explanation for the reduction of effect of repeated local anaesthetic injections. As the bicarbonate level falls, there is a migration of carbon dioxide from the cell, raising the intracellular pH. Replacement of the hydrochloride salt of the local anaesthetic by carbonated solutions induces rapid penetration of carbon dioxide into the nerve, causing a reduction of intraneural pH and promoting ionization of the drug intracellularly, where it is required. Carbonated solutions of local anaesthetics provide a more rapid and more profound block than comparable hydrochloride solutions.

Salicylate absorption is profoundly influenced by gastric pH. When acidity is increased, salicylates are less ionized and tend to be absorbed more quickly. However, decreased acidity in the stomach increases the solubility of salicylate, increasing the area for its absorption. The absorption half-time for unbuffered aspirin is 30 minutes, for buffered aspirin 20 minutes, and for aspirin solution a little less. Gastric emptying is reduced by antacids so that access to the large absorptive surface of the small intestine is delayed. Antacids also increase urinary excretion of the salicylates by increasing the ionization and preventing renal reabsorption. Alkalinization of the urine is an important method of treating salicylate poisoning.

Renal excretion

Excretion of drugs and metabolites by the kidney depends mainly upon their volume of distribution. If a drug is water-soluble and ionized (polar), it does not readily cross lipid membranes. It will be distributed only in the extracellular volume. It appears in the glomerular filtrate and will not be reabsorbed. Glomerular filtration rate is approximately 1% of the extracellular volume per minute so that the half-time of the exponential clearance of the ECF is 69 minutes (0.69 is the natural logarithm of 2). A lipid-soluble drug which crosses cell membranes is distributed throughout the total body water and would be reabsorbed by the tubules, so that the concentration in the urine is only that of plasma. The half-time of excretion, depending upon urine flow, could be about

20 days. A drug which is actively secreted into the urine by the renal tubules is cleared more quickly. Conversely, a drug which is dissolved in body fats or bound to tissue proteins has a greatly expanded volume of distribution, and the excretion of this drug depends almost entirely on transformation to more ionized metabolites. The degree of ionization of drugs depends upon the pK of the drug and the pH of the solution. Thus, acceleration of elimination of acids such as salicylates can be achieved by alkalinization of the urine, and of bases such as lignocaine by acidification.

Renal failure affects the elimination of drugs. The volume of distribution is altered by acidaemia, except where it is already extensive. Hepatic clearance of morphine is unaltered, but that of pethidine and fentanyl is increased. However, the metabolites of these drugs accumulate. One of the metabolites of pethidine — norpethidine — is a convulsant. Morphine glucuronides may be hydrolysed and reabsorbed because of passage through the gut, and may themselves accumulate to a concentration at which they, especially the 6-glucuronide, pass across the blood–brain barrier to achieve narcotic effect. Fentanyl metabolites have insignificant effects.

Hepatic factors

The liver has considerable reserve capacity, and biotransformation of drugs is not affected until hepatic injury is severe and widespread. In the newborn, hepatic function is not fully developed, and conjugation of bilirubin and morphine is incomplete. In hepatic cirrhosis and hepatitis, pethidine metabolism is reduced. Fentanyl metabolism has many pathways and is relatively spared in hepatic disease. Blood flow through the liver is a controlling factor in the biotransformation of most drugs. It is increased by beta-adrenergic drugs and decreased by alpha-adrenergic ones. Thus, it is decreased by a beta-blocker such as propranolol and by an alpha-sympathomimetic such as ephedrine. It is also decreased by the surgical planes of anaesthesia, by haemorrhage, and in shock. In all these conditions, the rate of biotransformation is decreased. This appears to be of no clinical significance in the case of morphine, fentanyl, or even pethidine, but the toxicity of lignocaine and other amide local anaesthetics and of paracetamol is increased.

The hepatic enzyme systems may be altered. Mention has already been made of the effect of carbon monoxide. Cimetidine may decrease liver blood flow, but its effects on opioids is mainly as an inhibitor of hepatic oxidative metabolism, which is the route of biotransformation of pethidine and one of those of fentanyl.

The microsomal enzyme systems are also subject to *enzyme induction*, e.g. induced synthesis of cytochrome P_{450} and cytochome P_{450} reductase, and proliferation of the endoplasmic reticulum. Phenobarbitone, a potent enzyme inducer, also increases hepatic blood and bile flow. Carbamazepine, although not an analgesic, is a drug of first choice for trigeminal, glossopharyngeal and post-herpetic neuralgia: it induces enzymes for the metabolism of itself and other drugs, and this mechanism may be responsible for the failure of prolonged therapy.

Severe hepatic disease and starvation lead to deficiency of proteins, including plasma proteins. This may lead to more unbound drug being available for membrane transfer and receptor occupancy. Aspirin and some other non-steroidal anti-inflammatory drugs (NSAIDs) compete with warfarin and phenytoin for the binding sites, and upset the balance of blood coagulation and increase phenytoin toxicity respectively. *In vitro*, the addition of pethidine to normal human plasma causes a displacement of previously administered bupivacaine. Clinical studies have not demonstrated that the sensitivity of patients with hepatic damage to pethidine is due to reduced plasma protein binding, and sensitivity to fentanyl (with 85% protein binding) is not increased in hepatic cirrhosis.

The sensitivity to orally administered drugs with significant first-pass metabolism is increased in those with liver disease, e.g. the potency of morphine will be increased by up to three times, and that of buprenorphine much more. Similarly, bypass of the liver by drugs in the plasma occurs in portal hypertension when portosystemic anastomoses are opened up. In liver damage, all drugs should be treated with caution. Postoperative analgesia is better treated with fentanyl or morphine than with pethidine, or with aspirin rather than paracetamol. An ester-type local anaesthetic is preferable to an amide-type, provided that the plasma cholinesterase levels are satisfactory and that the blood clotting factors are sufficient for the regional anaesthetic technique.

Table 13.2. Analgesic variability as a result of pharmacokinetic interactions of drugs.

Pharmacokinetic drug interactions

Absorption from the gut

Most drugs are absorbed in the small intestine. Basic drugs will be less ionized in the alkaline medium and will be soluble in the membrane of the gut wall. Even some acidic drugs such as aspirin are insoluble in the acid contents of the stomach and are absorbed principally from the jejunum and ileum. Some analgesics such as diflunisal and piroxicam are absorbed almost entirely from the stomach.

Absorption from the skin, muscle, rectum, and buccal cavity

Absorption is dependent on the regional blood flow. Vasoconstrictors applied with the drug reduce absorption, but drugs which cause generalized vasodilation or reduced cardiac output also reduce absorption because the regional distribution of blood to these areas is reduced in favour of that to more vital areas.

Distribution

A reduced cardiac output increases the proportion of blood flow to brain and heart. Drugs which act on these organs will be more potent when given intravenously in the presence of reduced cardiac output.

Biotransformation and excretion

Drugs may compete for enzymatic reduction, oxidation, conjugation, etc. Drugs may induce the synthesis of enzymes which biotransform themselves and other drugs. Drugs may increase or reduce the blood flow to organs of excretion (liver, kidneys, lungs). They may damage these organs and thereby potentiate the activities of other drugs.

Table 13.2. Continued.

Alteration of absorption	Interacting drugs	Analgesics affected	Mechanism
Delayed gastric emptying	Antacids, antimuscarinics	Paracetamol, aspirin[1] narcotic analgesics	Delays absorption of drugs, especially basic drugs, from the small intestine
Decreased gastric acidity	Antacids, buffers	Diflunisal, piroxicam	Reduces absorption of diflunisal, piroxicam; increases absorption of aspirin
Incomplete absorption from gut	Emetics, e.g. apomorphine, ipecacuanha	All oral preparations, especially enteric-coated capsules, morphine, buprenorphine	Used to induce vomiting in some cases of self-poisoning
	Purgatives, bulk and stimulant, e.g. ispaghula husk, senna		Hastens passage through small and large intestine; also decreases reabsorption of drugs which are excreted in the bile
Altered absorption from tissues	Vasoconstrictors, e.g. Adrenaline, felypressin	Local anaesthetics	Delays uptake by capillary blood but not by neural tissue
	Cardiovascular depressants, e.g. general anaesthetics, barbiturates, hypotensive agents	Intramuscular drugs Local anaesthetics	Delayed systemic uptake because blood flow diverted from muscles and skin to more vital organs
	Diuretics, e.g. frusemide	Local anaesthetics	Hypokalaemia reduces uptake by neural tissue
	Local anaesthetics, especially chloroprocaine, other acids[2]	Local anaesthetics, especially bupivacaine	Tissue acidosis reduces neural uptake: one mechanism of tachyphylaxis
	Rubifacients, e.g. capsaicin, chemical irritants	Parenteral analgesics Local anaesthetics	The inflammatory response decreases neural uptake but increases systemic uptake and toxicity
	Circulatory stimulants, e.g. isoprenaline, doxapram, thyroxine	All drugs	Improves cardiac output and tissue perfusion, thereby increasing uptake

Altered absorption/ excretion by the lungs	Circulatory stimulants	Nitrous oxide	Improves gas exchange and uptake of inhalational analgesic
	Circulatory depressants e.g. anaesthetics; ventilatory depressants, e.g. morphine	Trichlorethylene	Decreases gas exchange and reduces uptake
	Bronchodilators, e.g. salbutamol		May improve gas exchange by reducing airway resistance but also increase ventilatory dead space
Altered distribution	Circulatory depressants, e.g. anaesthetics, narcotics	All	Because of the contraction of the circulating volume and the greater proportion to the heart and brain, drugs entering the plasma have a greater effect on these organs
	Hyperhaemodynamic agents, e.g. thyroxine	All	Greater dilution of drug in circulating volume, therefore lower peak intensity of effect
Competition for protein binding sites	Warfarin, phenytoin. quinidine, propranolol	Aspirin, diflunisal, mefenamic acid *inter alia*	The drugs compete for the binding sites on the plasma proteins so that there is more free (effective) in the plasma
Altered biotransformation	Alcohol, adriamycin	Most analgesics, but *see* text	Capacity of hepatic enzyme pathways reduced; affects narcotic analgesics, simple analgesics, amide local anaesthetics; fentanyl less affected; nitrous oxide unaffected
Decreased hepatic blood flow	Alpha-adrenergic sympathomimetic amines; beta-adrenergic blockers; general anaesthetics; cimetidine	Narcotic analgesics, local anaesthetics	Principally affects drugs which have a high rate of metabolism, e.g. lignocaine

Table 13.2. *Continued.*

Alteration of absorption	Interacting drugs	Analgesics affected	Mechanism
Enzyme competition	Phenytoin, warfarin	Pethidine, salicylates but only in high dosage	Competition for enzymes *in vivo* is rare except when the metabolic process is already saturated as may occur in overdose
Enzyme inhibition	Carbon monoxide, as in tobacco smoking	Pethidine	By interference with cytochrome P_{450}, carbon dioxide blocks hepatic oxidation
	Monoamine oxidase inhibitors e.g. tranylcypromine, phenelzine, iproniazid, isocarboxazid	Narcotic analgesics	See Note 3
Excretion			
Increased alimentary excretion	Purgatives, glycerine suppositories	Entric-coated aspirin	Enteric-coated capsules may pass through unabsorbed
		Morphine, buprenorphine	The re-uptake of drugs excreted in the bile is reduced
		Rectal analgesics	The evacuation of drugs given rectally causes the amount absorbed to be less and unknown
Increased urine flow	Cardiac stimulants e.g. digoxin, thyroxine	Most analgesics	Improved renal blood flow and size of glomerular filtrate
	Renal artery dilation, e.g. low-dose dopamine; diuretics e.g. frusemide		Decreases tubular reabsorption

	vasoconstrictors e.g. noradrenaline, high-dose dopamine	constriction of renal arteries reduces filtration of drug from the plasma
	'inactive' metabolites may achieve active concentrations e.g. morphine 6-glucuronide	
Renal tubular damage	Most non-steroidal anti-inflammatory drugs, phenacetin; gentamycin	Oliguria or anuria
	Most analgesics	
Increased acidity of urine	Ammonium chloride; many sterilized infusates e.g. dextrose, saline	Although the urinary excretion of local anaesthetic is increased, the toxicity with the cells of the heart and brain is also increased
	Local anaesthetics, other bases	
Alkalinization of urine	Buffers and alkali, e.g. sodium bicarbonate	Increases ionization and thereby decreases reabsorption at the renal tubule
	Aspirin	

Notes

1 *See* introduction.

2 Increased acidity of tissues at the site of the local anaesthetic injection increases the degree of ionization of the anaesthetic and decreases its ability to penetrate the nerve membrane. Local anaesthetics in buffered solution (e.g. Ringer solution) equilibrated with carbon dioxide have decreased latency of onset, increased potency, increased duration, and greater degree of motor block. It is probable that carbon dioxide diffuses through the nerve membrane and increases the ionization of the local anaesthetic *inside* the cell. The active ion binds to the receptor and is also less able to diffuse out of the cell (ion trapping).

3 Monamine oxidase inhibitors act primarily extrahepatically. They interfere with the metabolism of monoamines like noradrenaline, dopamine, and 5-hydroxytryptamine. They interfere less with the effect of exogenously administered noradrenaline since the offset of action of this drug is because of uptake by the tissues rather than because of metabolism. They potentiate sympathomimetic amines such as ephedrine and phenylephrine and the hypertensive effect of the tricyclic antidepressants. The interaction with narcotic analgesics is less certain. They potentiate and alter the action of pethidine, possibly by inhibition of *N*-demethylation, such that it is increased and prolonged and may be accompanied by excitation and hyperpyrexic crises. This latter effect may be blocked by 5 hydroxytryptamine antagonists. Other narcotic analgesics are less affected, but are nonetheless potentiated and should be used with caution.

Summary

Pharmacokinetics describes the fate of drugs within the body. It includes absorption, distribution and binding to plasma proteins and tissues. It includes metabolism or biotransformation, excretion, and the way that these processes are altered by the acid–base balance, ventilation, disease, and other drugs. Its study has great practical relevance. It can explain, in part, the great variation of effect of drugs, and it can help to predict the individual patient response. It can be used to help make a choice of the best analgesic drug or method in any situation, and it can help to use that drug to its best advantage.

CHAPTER 14
What Next?

The relief of postoperative pain is developing and improving, but in some centres more than others. The relative safety, efficiency and advantages of newer techniques must be established, not only in centres of excellence and in high-dependency units, but in the more dimly lit, poorer staffed, general purpose wards that make up the environment of the majority of postoperative patients. Improvements must be not only desirable but feasible within the staffing and financial budget of the hospital. Savings in human suffering, morbidity, mortality and duration of postoperative stay and/or convalescence must be identifiable. It is the duty of those with the means of improving the postoperative care of the patient not only to lead the way, but to make it possible for others to follow.

Some developments are already established but are confined to a few centres. Others are identifiable but are either not available or are too costly (in money or time) for general use.

Equipment

There have been many welcome developments of equipment which increase the safety or efficacy of postoperative analgesia. In many cases the new equipment is so expensive that routine adoption is improbable. In some, the intrinsic cost of the materials and manufacture is great. In others, the cost of materials is little more than that which is currently available, but the reduced volume of manufacture renders the cost per item disproportionately high. In the latter case, it is to be hoped that more widespread use and a responsible pricing policy will allow the price per item to fall and the equipment to be adopted universally.

The commonly used epidural cannulae are those with closed ends and side-holes, the most proximal of which may be 1.8 cm from the tip. The cannulae are made from Teflon, polyethylene, or polyurethane (with or without plasticizers). They are flexible but almost inelastic in the long axis. Movements of the patient's trunk cause the cannula to move in and out through the skin puncture-incision, encouraging inflammation, epithelialization, and infection. The small side-holes become blocked with fibrin relatively quickly (sometimes within two postoperative days) and movements may cause the proximal side-hole to lie outside the epidural space. An implantation-grade silicone rubber catheter, yielding along its longitudinal axis, and with a terminal orifice, is commercially available in combination with an implantable epidural reservoir or pump. This could be made available (without reservoir) for prolonged percutaneous use at little extra cost.

Subcutaneous cannulae. Infusion of local anaesthetics into the wound must be slow and distributed evenly along the wound. A thin cannula is required (about 18 swg) with a Luer-lock hub, a closed tip, and with side-holes every 0.5 cm for 30–40 cm of its length.

Nerve blockade. With the exception of infiltration anaesthesia, nerve blockade should not be performed with hypodermic needles. These have long bevels with knife-sharp edges. They can cut the nerve sheath or the axon, leading to neuromata. *A spinal-type needle*, which has a short bevel with unsharpened sides, should be used instead. Hopefully, a manufacturer will realize the potential size of the market of peripheral nerve blockade and, since the continuing cost of production of a short-bevel needle is no more than that of hypodermic needles, will produce such a disposable needle at a comparable price.

Pain and paraesthesia should not be sought, as this may result in nerve entry and damage. It is suggested that a *nerve stimulator* be used. One electrode is connected to the needle and one, the indifferent electrode, attached to the skin at a distant site. It provides a charge maximal at the tip of the needle. The sensation evoked increases as the nerve trunk is approached. Although purpose-designed insulated needles exist (e.g. Top-pole), a steel spinal needle is satisfactory for most purposes. The use of a nerve stimulator increases the accuracy of needle placement near peripheral nerves and the reliability of the anaesthesia

Monitoring ventilatory rate and pattern is time-consuming to the nurse and, since adequate light is required, disturbing to the patient at night. *Respiratory monitoring devices* exist (e.g. Respitrace) but, at present, they are expensive, bulky, and restricting. Hopefully, telemetry of the pulmonary impedence, nasopharyngeal temperatures, or carbon dioxide expiration will provide a more practical solution. The resurgence of interest of feedback modulation of anaesthesia and analgesia during operation may extend to the postoperative period.

Manpower and resources

Analgesic teams

Already, in a few institutions, a team of medical and/or nursing staff, expert and experienced in pain relief, is available for help and advice. The team can help those whose conditions or existing therapy present special risks or problems, those whose pain appears resistant to routine therapy, or those who develop intolerable side-effects. Pain can change in character, site, or implication and may be due to compression of nerves themselves. A diagnostic and nerve blockade service can be provided.

Intermediate-term recovery rooms

Improved monitoring, diagnosis of pain, and application of pain-relieving procedures are enabled by the provision of continuous recovery wards which are open for 24 hours each day. They receive, from the operating theatres, patients who would benefit from surgical and anaesthetic management for longer than is available in a short-term recovery room, but of less complexity than is available in an intensive therapy unit.

Such a ward could minimize the disturbance on the general ward and provide a level of lighting and trained staffing which would allow adequate monitoring. Those units which are adjacent to the theatres and intensive therapy unit appear to be most efficient and can provide immediate analgesia, etc. Many patients undergoing minor or peripheral surgery would not need these facilities but, to others, immediate access to pain relief, infusion pumps, suction, monitoring, bladder-washouts, etc. is more important on the day of operation than the flowers, get-well cards, and grapes, which are of much psychological value later in the recovery process.

Techniques

The use of spinally applied opioids is an example of a technique with known advantages, especially for thoracic and abdominal pain, which is not yet widespread. In some centres, it is confined to the high-dependency units, in others it is not used at all. It cannot be said to be completely safe, yet our experience of six years' use in the general postoperative wards indicates that, provided certain safeguards are maintained, it is less productive of respiratory depression than bolus intravenous or intramuscular injections of opioids. The safeguards, as explained more fully in Chapter 11, are that a lipid-soluble opioid is used (e.g. diamorphine) and that following a small bolus dose it is infused slowly by means of an accurate pump, such that the opioid is taken up by only the appropriate spinal segments, Ventilation is monitored hourly until six hours after the infusion has been discontinued, and the infusion is stopped if the ventilation slows below 12 breaths per minute or becomes irregular.

Hypnosis, i.e. the induction of a hypersuggestible state of relaxation, has not, so far, been described in this book. Post operative analgesia by this means requires considerable skill and practice; it is not suitable for all patients; it requires pretreatment, in almost every case, preoperatively; and the degree of pain relief is unpredictable. Recently, M.J. Griffiths and his colleagues have demonstrated (data not yet published) that the suggestible state of hypnosis is associated with specific changes in the electroenecephalogram, and that this state can be reproduced (or its achievement can be enhanced) by the inhalation of very low concentrations of either nitrous oxide or enflurane. This state can be demonstrated by the subjects conforming to post-hynotic suggestions. Light planes of anaesthesia are distinguishable from this state both by the encephalogram and by the lack of effect of suggestion. If confirmed, these aids would enhance the speed and predictability of analgesia by hypnoidal suggestion.

Electroanaesthesia and electroanalgesia are not recent innovations, but, with the exception of transcutaneous electrical nerve stimulation, are rarely used in the postoperative period. Dorsal column stimulation is used mainly for chronic pain, via electrodes implanted percutaneously under radiographic control, or under direct vision at operation. Inhibition of pain from a limb or segment of the body can also be achieved by transcutaneous stimulation of a subcutaneous nerve trunk or by the implantation of suitable electrodes onto deeper nerve trunks or within neurovascular sheaths (Long & Hagfors 1975).

Drugs

Local anaesthesia

The requirement for a longer acting local anaesthetic agent is superficially obvious. The blocking of painful stimuli while healing occurs would appear to be of unalloyed benefit. Yet infusion techniques already exist and are not used more frequently partly because of the incidence of complications and disadvantages. There is no reason to suppose that a long-acting agent would produce pain relief or even sensory loss without a concomitant loss of function or protection. Loss of tactile sense or proprioception of the legs would still be associated with enforced immobility, sympathetic block with postural hypotension or loss of heat. Yet such an agent would have considerable value if it could be confined, say, to intercostal nerves whose loss of function is of limited significance, rather than be applied to the paravertebral or epidural space, where uncontrolled spread could cause prolonged difficulty and danger. There is the additional risk that prolonged loss of sensation in one part of the receptor field of a spinal nerve can cause abnormal sensitivity in another, such as muscle pain, phantom limb, sympathetically mediated pain, etc., or in the receptor fields of adjacent nerves.

The further elucidation of the mechanism by which capsaicin is able to block small sensory nerves might eventually produce a local agent for use in postoperative pain that lacks the disadvantages of current local anaesthetics. The topical application of bradykinin receptor antagonists is another possibility for local therapy.

Regional analgesics

Spinally applied opioids can achieve effective regional analgesia but at the risk of ventilatory depression. The alpha$_2$ agonist clonidine can also be given spinally to produce effective regional analgesia but may cause somnolence and hypotension. Subanalgesic doses of clonidine and morphine have an additive analgesic action (p. 87), and the combination of spinal opioid and alpha$_2$ agonist may prove to give effective analgesia at less risk.

Systemic analgesics

Considerable space has been given to drugs under development in the relevant chapters earlier in the book. It is true to say, however, that the advance in this field that will be of most benefit is the provision of analgesia coupled with minimal side-effects. Only time and clinical experience will tell us whether this is likely to result from the use of potent cyclo-oxygenase inhibitors or of selective kappa opioids. Should these strategies prove to be blind alleys, then the current expansion in neurobiology, particularly in the field of neuropeptides, will produce many more leads for the medicinal chemist and pharmacologist to follow in the search for the ideal analgesic.

APPENDIX I
Drug Interactions

Endogenous ligands (pharmacologically active substances) can produce specific actions by combining with a receptor, and by being released and destroyed at the site of the receptor. Substances which are released into the bloodstream, and drugs which are taken orally or given parenterally, are active throughout the body and must be expected to have a range of actions. Drugs given concurrently may interact at the same receptor, or at different receptors, to produce a change in a common pathway, or have effects which are similar or opposite.

Drugs can compete for binding with a receptor. At low doses, the more agonist drug given, the greater the effect, but at higher doses the increase in effect becomes less with each incremental dose until a maximum effect is reached. The amount of drug required to produce this is inversely proportional to its potency, and the magnitude of the maximal effect is related to its efficacy. Additionally, the forces which bind the drug to the receptor vary in strength. If a drug binds to a receptor to produce a maximal effect, it is called a full agonist. If it produces less than the maximal effect, it is a partial agonist. If a partial agonist competes for the same receptor as a full agonist, it can function as an antagonist. If it binds with the receptor in competition with an agonist but has no intrinsic effect, it is called a pure antagonist. Potency has little clinical relevance *per se* unless the drug is so weak and insoluble that the bulk of drug to be administered is an embarassment. Fentanyl is 1000 times as potent as pethidine, but 10 000 times as expensive.

Potency is related not only to the affinity of the drug for the receptor, but its availability to the receptor in terms of absorption, transfer, and distribution. Drugs may therefore also interact with each other with regard to absorption, binding, distribution, membrane transfer, metabolism, and excretion. The dose which produces the maximum effect at one receptor may not be that which is maximally effective at another, e.g. maximal pentazocine analgesia is probably produced by 30–60 mg/70 kg; doses in excess of this increase the incidence of hallucinations.

Common pathways of action are exemplified by the synergism of morphine and other narcotics. The ventilatory depressive effect of morphine is antagonized by pain and anxiety and other powerful stimuli via the reticular activating system. Local anaesthesia, anxiolysis, and narcosis reduce the stimulation and potentiate the ventilatory depression.

Drug synergism or antagonism may be the result of two similar actions at unrelated sites, e.g. myocardial depression by lignocaine and beta-adrenergic blocking drugs, one acting on the myocardium and the other primarily on the neural inflow. Further potentiation of lignocaine by beta-blockers occurs because the latter decrease hepatic blood flow and reduce lignocaine biotransformation.

Table of drug interactions.

Drug	Effects
INTERACTION WITH OPIOIDS	
Absorption	
Metoclopramide	Increases absorption from oral administration: drug action opposed by the opioid
Purgatives	Decrease absorption of rectal or oral drug, especially slow-release preparation: drug action opposed by the opioid
Elimination	
Beta-blockers	Reduce hepatic blood flow and decrease rate of biotransformation: little clinical significance in man
Cimetidine	Reduces hepatic blood flow, also decreases hepatic oxidation — decreases clearance of fentanyl and pethidine
Tricyclic antidepressants	Inhibit metabolism of methadone
Chlorpromazine	Increases proportion of norpethidine from pethidine: this is a convulsant
Monoamine oxidase inhibitors	Blocks mixed hepatic oxidation: combined with pethidine may cause hyperpyrexia, respiratory depression, tachycardia and

Drug interactions Continued.

Drug	Effects
Monoamine oxidase inhibitors *continued*	hypotension. May cause hyper- or hypotension with other opioids
Tobacco	Biotransformation increased because of liver enzyme induction; may also cause cross-tolerance at cellular level because of changes in cyclic AMP-ase
Phenobarbitone, other barbiturates, carbamazepine	Induction of hepatic enzymes: increase rate of biotransformation of opioids
Rifampicin, an antituberculous drug	Accelerates metabolism of methadone and may precipitate withdrawal

Pharmacodynamics

Drug	Effects
Phenothiazines, benzodiazepines, and other narcotics/sedatives	Increased narcosis and ventilatory depression in response to carbon dioxide and lack of response to airway obstruction
Some phenothiazines, e.g. chlorpromazine, promethazine, and barbiturates	Inhibit analgesia despite increased narcosis
Hydroxyzine (antihistamine drug)	Increases analgesia (may act at opioid receptor)
Amphetamines in small doses	Enhance analgesia
Physostigmine, neostigmine, tetrahydroaminoacrine	Enhance analgesia — mechanism may be a central cholinergic effect
Non-depolarizing muscle relaxants	Opioids increase duration of effect because of lack of respiratory drive. Muscle relaxants may reduce postoperative pain — *see* Chapter 1
General anaesthetics	Synergistic narcotic action. Most opioid agonists reduce minimum anaesthetic concentration (MAC). Partial agonists reduce MAC much less
Alpha-adrenergic blocking drugs	Inhibition of compensatory vasoconstriction — postural hypotension increased after most opioids

Drug Interactions *Continued.*

Drug	Effects
Xanthine and related compounds, e.g. coffee tea, cocoa, cola	Release opioid-induced contraction of smooth muscle in intestine and biliary tract and also antagonize opioid-induced inhibition of longitudinal muscle of intestinal tract

INTERACTION WITH NON-STEROIDAL ANTI-INFLAMMATORY DRUGS AND PARACETAMOL

Absorption

Drug	Effects
Antacids	Delay gastric emptying and reduce acidity: increase solubility and absorption of aspirin, indomethacin, naproxen, and enteric-coated phenylbutazone and aspirin. Elimination of aspirin increased. Reduced absorption of diflunisal
Alcohol	Increases incidence of gastric bleeding
Cimetidine, ranitidine	Reduces acid secretion and protects gastric mucosa from aspirin-induced ulceration
Metoclopramide	Speeds gastric emptying and absorption of paracetamol. Reduces absorption of diflunisal and (?) piroxicam.

Protein binding

NSAIDs are bound extensively to plasma proteins (paracetamol up to 20%, salicylates 8%, piroxicam 99%). They compete with other drugs for these sites. The concurrent use of these and other bound drugs leads to the unbound portion of both drugs being increased and potentiation of both drugs.

Drug	Effects
Warfarin and phenindione	Increase anticoagulant effect with aspirin, phenylbutazone; probable potentiation with diflunisal, mefenamic acid, piroxicam, and indomethacin. Potentiation with high or prolonged dosage of ibuprofen and paracetamol (because of hepatic enzyme induction)
Heparin	Potentiated by aspirin
Sulphonylurea hypoglycaemic agents	Potentiation, especially with aspirin and phenylbutazone
Methotrexate	Potentiated, especially with aspirin and phenylbutazone

Drug Interactions *Continued.*

Drug	Effects
Tricyclic antidepressants, barbiturates, phenytoin, sulphonamides	All potentiated
Thyroxine	Potentiated
Vitamin C in high dose	Potentiates NSAIDs
NSAIDs	Aspirin displaces indomethacin and naproxen from plasma proteins
Probenecid	Plasma concentration increased by indomethacin
Pharmacodynamic interactions	
Antihypertensive drugs	Reduced effect with indomethacin and phenylbutazone
Beta-blockers	Antagonism of antihypertensive effect by indomethacin
ADH, pitressin	Paracetamol and indomethacin enhance effect of ADH by inhibition of the ADH-stimulated production of prostaglandin, thereby preventing negative feedback
Spironolactone	Diuretic effect inhibited by aspirin.
Probenecid	Uricosuric effect inhibited by aspirin. Synergism with phenylbutazone
Penicillin	Aspirin blocks transfer of penicillin from CSF to blood
Biotransformation	
Insulin	Inactivation inhibited by phenylbutazone
Anticoagulants	Chronic paracetamol administration induces hepatic breakdown and slightly increases prothrombopenic effect

INTERACTION WITH
LOCAL ANAESTHETICS

Adrenaline, felypressin octopressin	Reduce systemic absorption, lower toxicity, prolong action

Drug interactions Continued.

Drug	Effects
Carbonated solutions	Increase uptake by neural tissue
Dextran	Prolongs action — see Chapter 3
Penicillin	Procaine can conjugate with other drugs and prolong their absorption
Biotransformation	
Neostigmine	Inhibits plasma cholinesterase — potentiation
Methylprednisolone and dexamethasone	Decrease plasma cholinesterase
Suxamethonium	Competes for plasma cholinesterase — rarely clinically significant
Beta-adrenergic blockers	Reduce liver blood flow and amide-type metabolism — potentiation
Phenobarbitone	This and other enzyme inducers increase the metabolism of the amide-type local anaesthetics
General anaesthetics, hypotensive agents	Decrease regional blood flow to liver, decrease amide-type metabolism — potentiation
Amide–ester mixtures	Amide-type local anaesthetics inhibit hydrolysis, ester-type have low pH and cause tachyphylaxis of amide
Cimetidine	Decreases liver blood flow and (also) inhibits metabolism of amides — potentiation
Plasma protein binding	
Phenytoin, quinidine, pethidine	Displace amides from plasma protein: bupivacaine and etidocaine most affected
Pharmacodynamics	
General anaesthesia (low dose), barbiturates	Increase sedative effects of local anaesthetics (except cocaine); increase threshold for convulsions, increase cardiac depressant effects
Tricyclic antidepressants	These increase the amount of 5-hydroxytryptophan in the cerebrum and increase sensitivity to convulsions

Drug interactions *Continued.*

Drug	Effects
D-Tubocurarine	Elevates convulsive threshold
Non-depolarizing muscle relaxants	Decrease requirement because local anaesthetics have a stabilizing effect on the post-junctional membrane and have a central effect on muscle relaxation
Beta-adrenergic blockers	Potentiate myocardial depression and bradycardia
Calcium antagonists: nifedipine, verapamil	Synergistic myocardial depression and bradycardia
INTERACTIONS WITH KETAMINE	
Barbiturates	Chemically incompatible — precipitation
All narcotics, e.g. barbiturates, narcotic analgesics, benzodiazepines	Prolonged recovery
Morphine	Decreased incidence of emergence phenomena and hyperhaemodynamic reactions
INTERACTIONS WITH NEFOPAM	
Monoamine oxidase inhibitors	Potentiation
Sympathomimetics	Effects additive
Anticholinergic drugs	Effects additive

APPENDIX II
Analgesic Overdose and its Treatment

Postoperatively, analgesic overdosage is less common than underdosage, but it can be lethal, and all areas of postoperative care should have the means and skill to treat overdosage of the analgesics used.

Overdosage may be the result of:

1 An error in prescribing because of faulty knowledge or memory.
2 An error of judgement of the patient's size or condition.
3 An error in reading the prescription, the time, or the drug label, or in identifying the patient.
4 The dose may be inappropriate for the route: for example, a dose intended to be given intramuscularly may be given into a vein; the tourniquet may deflate during an intravenous regional injection of local anaesthetic; a bolus or part of a bolus of local anaesthetic drug, intended for the stellate ganglion or a field block of the tonsillar bed, may be injected into a cerebral artery. In each case, the peak effect is much greater than that intended although the total amount of drug is the same.
5 The absorption or distribution of the drug may be abnormal: the absorption or oral morphine may be delayed until after a second dose is given; in cases of hypotension and shock, regional blood flow is altered so that absorption of an intramuscular or subcutaneous dose is delayed and the distribution of an intravenous dose is more predominantly to the heart and brain than is usual. Passage across inflamed membrane barriers may be increased, as in the absorption of local anaesthetics in infected sites or the increased effect of morphine in cases of meningitis. In the newborn, the blood—brain barrier is underdeveloped and morphine has an increased effect.
6 The dose may be inappropriate for the condition of the patient. If hepatic or renal function is altered, the biotransformation and excretion of the drug may be reduced, so that accumulation occurs. These functions may be altered so that active metabolites

Analgesic Overdose and Treatment 239

are increased in production or are reduced in elimination, e.g. the excitatory effects of nor-pethidine or the increased effect of morphine 6-glucuronide in patients with decreased renal function. The patient's condition of debility, e.g. septicaemia, acidosis, atherosclerosis, hyperthyroidism, etc., may render him more susceptible to the action of the analgesic.

7 Drugs given concurrently may potentiate the action of the analgesic or may have a toxic effect similar to that of the analgesic (*see* Appendix I).

8 The condition of the patient may change following administration of the analgesic. For example, even if the dose of opiate given was suitable for the condition of the patient and appropriate to relieve the pain at the time of administration, circumstances may change such that the analgesic medication is in excess of that required to combat the pain. Certain stimulating events, such as physiotherapy, tracheal toilet, are short-lived, some pains such as convulsive pains or colic are severe but remit spontaneously, or the wound pain may be relieved by local anaesthetic techniques when opioid medication seems ineffective. With the relief of pain or the cessation of stimulation, opioids become relatively more narcotic, and the patient may lapse into stupor and ventilatory depression.

9 Where the analgesic is self-administered, either at home or as part of a patient-controlled analgesic technique, failure of the drug to act as quickly or as effectively as expected may lead to excessive repetition of administration and to acute or chronic poisoning.

The effects of overdosage can be prevented or reduced by *monitoring* and *early treatment*. *Further absorption* should be prevented or delayed. The absorption of orally administered drugs can be reduced many hours after ingestion by vomiting, gastric lavage, and the use of charcoal. In the fully conscious patient, when no irritant substances have been ingested, vomiting can be induced by ipecacuanha or by apomorphine. The latter is given slowly intravenously until the first sensation of nausea is experienced. The injection is stopped, vomiting follows shortly afterwards, and the sense of nausea declines rapidly as the drug is redistributed. Should nausea or vomiting persist in spite of an empty stomach, the effect can be reversed by a *small* bolus of droperidol given intravenously. Alternatively, gastric lavage should be performed, in a head-down position, using a large-bore gastric tube introduced through the mouth. Charcoal (e.g. Medicoal) effectively adsorbs many drugs and toxins and improves the elimination of the drug. If the patient is not fully conscious, if there is any reduction of the cough or gagging reflex, or if any irritant substances have been ingested (e.g. methanol, bleach, peanuts), the patient should be intubated before gastric lavage.

Drugs given by infusion should be stopped and the absorption of drugs given by subcutaneous or intramuscular injection can be delayed temporarily by the use of a tourniquet.

The active proportion of a drug can be altered by the adjustment of the acidity of the plasma and alteration of the regional blood flow. Biotransformation and elimination can be controlled by alteration of the acid—base balance and adjustment of the cardiac output and the hepatic and renal blood flow, and, if necessary, by the use of peritoneal haemodialysis and exchange transfusions (infants).

General resuscitation measures include maintenance of the airway, adequacy of ventilation and gas exchange, cardiac output, blood pressure, and tissue perfusion. If possible, specific antagonists to the drugs or to the mediators of effect should be used. Replacement of the system poisoned or of the means of drug destruction may be possible (infusion of liver cells, renal transplants, etc.).

Opioids

Recognition

Mild to moderate overdosage is usually diagnosed by slow, deep ventilations, reduction of consciousness and pin-point pupils. Hypotension is predominantly postural, unless the level of the blood pressure was previously maintained by pain. However, other forms of ventilatory dysfunction may be seen instead, for instance periodic ventilation which has periods of overtly normal ventilation, or deep ventilation interspersed with periods of apnoea.

More severe ventilatory dysfunction is associated with slow *shallow* ventilation, reduction of the minute volume, and an increase of the carbon dioxide tension. Consciousness is further reduced, even on stimulation, and the airway may become occluded.

Severe overdosage is associated with ventilatory arrest, coma, dilated pupils, hypotension and pulmonary oedema.

Treatment

The airway should be supported, and artifical ventilation instituted if necessary. In all cases, except for severe overdosage with pulmonary oedema, or for those with an intrathecal or epidural bolus of opioids, the hypotension should be improved by head-down tilting. The hypotension could be improved further by infusions of fluid or by the use of a vasoconstrictor, but the more specific treatment is by intravenous naloxone. This is given in boluses of 0.1 mg every one or two minutes until a satisfactory response is obtained. If after 2 mg the ventilatory depression is not improved, it is unlikely to be due to opioid overdosage, (but *see below* with regard to buprenorphine). Ten milligrams of naloxone have been given as a single bolus without obvious side-effects, but high doses may cause twitching or convulsions. Naloxone has been used successfully in the treatment of shock owing to anaphylaxis, sepsis, and haemorrhage (Gullo & Romano 1983). Naloxone is less successful against the kappa agonists such as pentazocine, and larger doses may have to be used. The binding of buprenorphine to the mu receptor is greater than that of naloxone, so that although naloxone can prevent the analgesia and ventilatory depression of buprenorphine it cannot reliably be used to treat it. Respiratory depression because of buprenorphine overdose should be treated with ventilatory support and a respiratory stimulant such as doxapram. This latter is given as a very slow intravenous bolus of 1 mg per kg body weight, followed by careful monitoring and an infusion of approximately 2 mg per minute, depending on response. It is a general stimulant, and tachycardia and hypertension may require treatment with adrenergic-blocking drugs; bronchodilators and muscle spasmolytics may also be needed.

Respiratory depression following the use of spinal opioids may also be treated by intravenous naloxone. This may have to be repeated every 40−50 minutes, but there is the further advantage that the regional analgesia is usually maintained while the central ventilatory depression is reversed.

Recently three cases of delayed cardiovascular depression have been reported, associated with intravenous nalbuphine when used in combination with other central nervous system depressants (Lawrie & Drake 1985). All cases were treated successfully with naloxone and confirmatory evidence of this complication is awaited.

Non-steroidal anti-inflammatory drugs

Although paracetamol is an antipyretic analgesic drug, it is not anti-inflammatory, nor is it an inhibitor of peripheral cyclo-oxygenase, and it is considered later.

Many of the NSAIDs uncouple oxidative phosphorylation and increase metabolism, the formation of carbon dioxide, and the consumption of oxygen. All are predominantly bound to plasma proteins and all are cyclo-oxygenase inhibitors in the tissues and in platelets.

Chronic intoxication can occur with regular moderate intake which fully occupies the binding sites and which exceeds the capacity for biotransformation and elimination. Acute or chronic toxicity may be caused by the concurrent administration of drugs which share the same binding site. Chronic toxicity can be achieved by self-administration for tension headaches, arthralgia, and rheumatic conditions. Postoperatively, overdosage is not so common as with the opioids but may occur if these drugs are used for pain for which they are inappropriate. Very high plasma levels may be found after rectal administration of indomethacin and intramuscular injections of diclofenac. Life-threatening toxicity is sometimes achieved by the in-patient or out-patient with that intention.

Recognition

Toxicity of the anti-inflammatory drugs may present with bleeding from the gastrointestinal or renal tracts, or haemopoietic reactions such as neutropenia, thrombocytopenia, and aplastic anaemia. Mild to moderate chronic overdosage is recognized by headache, dizziness, ringing in the ears, partial deafness, diminished sight, mental confusion, drowsiness, sweating, thirst, and nausea.

Acute severe toxicity is characterized initially by hyperventilation, restlessness, incoherence, vertigo, tremor, delirium, hallucinations, convulsions, and coma. Nausea is common, Dehydration and acid–base upset occur. The blood sugar may be altered, but both hyperglycaemia and hypoglycaemia, especially in young children, can present. The acid—base state depends upon the duration and severity of the toxicity. Initially there is a respiratory alkalosis due to the centrally stimulated hyperventilation. Later central stimulation is replaced by depression and, at the same time, a compensatory metabolic acidosis develops. Finally there is medullary depression together with a respiratory and a metabolic acidosis.

Treatment

The plasma level of the drug in question should be estimated, as should the status of acid—base and electrolyte balance. Unless treatment is very delayed, it should be initially directed towards preventing any further absorption of the drug. If the patient is fully conscious, vomiting should be induced. If not, gastric lavage and administration of activated charcoal is performed, following intubation of the trachea. The hyperthermia and dehydration is treated next by sponging and cooling combined with intravenous fluids, which should contain bicarbonate. The bicarbonate corrects the metabolic acidosis, shifts salicylate from the brain to the plasma, and hastens urinary excretion. (Too rapid infusion of bicarbonate may cause pulmonary oedema.) The ketosis and hypoglycaemia should be corrected by intravenous administration of glucose and, if necessary, insulin and potassium. The latter may be necessary since, as the acidosis is corrected, there is a shift of potassium from the extracellular to the intracellular space. If shock or hypotension is present, transfusion of plasma or human plasma protein fraction will be necessary, and, if haemorrhagic phenomena predominate, transfusion should be with whole blood. Forced alkaline diuresis is more effective than alkalinization alone, and in very severe cases exchange transfusion or haemo- or peritoneal dialysis may be required.

Paracetamol

Chronic overdosage of paracetamol may lead to hepatic damage and very occasionally to neutropenia, leucopenia and pancytopenia. It may also lead to prolonged coagulation of the blood in those on oral anticoagulant therapy, because of induced synthesis of the hepatic microsomal enzymes. However, primary toxicity can be due to acute overdosage of as little as 10 g of paracetamol, especially when taken with alcohol or other drugs which interfere with hepatic metabolism. Overdosage leads to hepatic necrosis, renal tubular necrosis, and hypoglycaemic coma. Because of its advertised safety, paracetamol toxicity is becoming more common. Furthermore, hepatic damage may not be noticeable immediately, but only after 2–6 days, and the only early signs are nausea and vomiting. Later, jaundice, coagulation disorders, and raised transaminases and lactic dehydrogenase develop. The best indicator that hepatic damage will occur is the half-life of paracetamol: hepatic necrosis is likely if the half-life is greater than 4 hours, and coma is likely if it is greater than 12. The plasma concentration of paracetamol is not as good an indicator, but serious hepatic damage is associated with a concentration of 300 mg/l at 4 hours after ingestion. Encephalopathy is also likely if the bilirubin exceeds 40 mg/l during the first five days.

Treatment

Paracetamol is not absorbed in the stomach, and further absorption can be reduced by induction of vomiting if the patient is conscious, or by intubation if the patient is unconscious, both followed by gastric lavage and administration of activated charcoal, 50 g in water, repeated at intervals. Forced alkaline diuresis is ineffective for paracetamol elimination. Haemodialysis has been advocated for all those whose paracetamol level is 120 mg/l at 4 hours after ingestion, but most authorities would suggest the use of acetylcysteine or methionine. Both act by replacing depleted stores of glutathione in the liver. Acetylcysteine can be given intravenously or orally. The dose is 150 mg/kg as an infusion over 15 minutes, followed by 70 mg/kg every four hours for three days. Methionine is given orally in a dose of 2.5 g in an adult followed by a further dose of 2.5 g four-hourly for the next 12 hours, and thereafter depending on the paracetamol concentration.

Local anaesthetics

The diagnosis and treatment of toxicity of local anaesthetics are described on p. 150.

APPENDIX II
Acute and Chronic Pain

	Acute pain	Chronic pain
Benefit	Promotes withdrawal from harm and rest during healing	None
Nociception	Direct result of applied stimulus	Often self-perpetuating
Severity	Related mainly to strength of stimulus	Only partially related to noxious stimulus
Behaviour	Usually appropriate to noxious stimulus	Often inappropriate to severity of stimulus
Mood	Anxiety	Depressed: increasing fatigue/irritability
Time-course	Improves with time	Does not improve with time
Autonomic changes	Related to sympathetic stimulation: Less persistalsis Increased ventilation and oxygen consumption Increased pulse rate and arterial pressures and cardiac work General peripheral vasoconstriction, but increased perfusion at the site of injury or inflammation Pupillary dilation and sweating	Pulse may be slow in conjunction with depression Hyperventilation may persist, leading to low plasma bicarbonate concentration Vasoconstriction of painful part, which is cold and pale: sympathetic dystrophic signs may be present[1]
Sleep pattern	Refreshing, occurs in spite of pain	Onset of sleep delayed; frequent awakening; fatigue persists in spite of sleep
Effect of antidepressants	Adrenaline-uptake inhibitors, e.g. desimipramine, are analgesic	Analgesic response to those which inhibit the uptake of serotonin, e.g. amitriptyline

Appendix III

Effect of attitude of attendants[2]	Analgesia enhanced by sympathy	Sympathy reinforces the pain behavioural patterns[2]

Notes

1 Sympathetic dystrophy is characterized by cold, pallor, swelling, and alteration of the growth of hair and nails of the injured part and of the surrounding area. Excessive vascular responses occur following dependence or changes in temperature. Weakness and loss of function occur, and rarefaction of bone may occur. Pain is evoked by non-noxious stimuli such as touching, and the sensation itself may be altered (allodynia). Pain may be constant and increased by cold, damp, stress, and other changes which cause release of noradrenaline. A similar condition is erythrodynia. The skin may be warm or cold or vary widely from one to the other; it may even show signs of ischaemia. The vascular changes are similar to those described above. The threshold of pain caused by heat is lowered so much that pain may be induced during warm weather, in bed at night, or in warm establishments such as hospitals. The victim may be able to control the pain only by immersing the part in water or ice.

2 Attendants in this context include the family, friends, and acquaintances, as well as the whole health care team (doctors, nurses, social workers, physiotherapists). Furthermore, the patient will seek those exhibiting the most sympathy, reinforcing the pain syndrome and leading to rejection and resentment of those who adopt a more realistic attitude, or those whose sympathy becomes diluted.

Glossary

Algogen A chemical substance that produces pain
Anaesthesia (anaesthetic) The absence of feeling or sensation
Analgesia The absence of pain
Analgesic (analgetic) Pertaining to analgesia; a drug which reduces pain
Caudally Towards the tail
Cephalad Towards the head
Cogener (congener) A member of the same kind or class
Denier One who denies: specifically in the preoperative period, one who denies that external events have importance or implications
Dynorphin Member of a family of endogenous opioid peptides
Embolus An intravascular mass, carried by the bloodstream from its point of origin
Enkephalin Naturally occurring pentapeptide opioid
Hyperpolarization Raising the membrane potential making the neurone less excitable
Ligand Any substance which combines with a receptor. The ligand−receptor complex may produce an effect (agonism) or may produce no effect (antagonism) but inhibit further binding by other substances
Lobotomize Lit. to cut a lobe — refers to incising a lobe of the brain: prefrontal leucotomy interrupts the frontothalamic projections; cingulotomy or amygdalotomy is more selective and causes fewer adverse personality changes
Modality Sensation, i.e. pain, touch, warmth etc., in the context of dorsal horn processing
Narcotic Pertaining to narcosis, a state of central nervous system depression. Used in the U.S.A. to denote drugs with addictive liability
NSAID Non-steroidal anti-inflammatory drug; this group of drugs includes all the cyclo-oxygenase (prostaglandin synthetase)

inhibitors with the exception of paracetamol and new agents that act on CNS cyclo-oxygenase

Opioids All substances acting at opioid receptors

Pharmacodynamics The consideration of the effect of drugs on the organism — sometimes interchangeable with pharmacology

Pharmacokinetics The consideration of the movement of drugs within an organism; it includes the absorption, distribution, binding, biotransformation and excretion of drugs

p.r.n. *Pro re nata*, literally 'according to circumstances'; drugs given p.r.n. are given on patient demand or as they are shown to be required

Pro-drug A substance which has little or no action on the body itself, but which is broken down or biotransformed into active ligand

Prostanoid Substance related to prostaglandins

Pseudounipolar neurone One with a single process which then branches in two directions

Thromboprophylaxis Measures taken to prevent clotting

References

Alexander J. & Black A.M.S. (1984) Comparing extradural and i.v. diamorphine and buprenorphine after abdominal surgery. *British Journal of Anaesthesia* **56**, 1283−4.
Alexander J.I. & Hull M.G.R. (1987) Abdominal pain after laparoscopy: the value of a gas drain. *British Journal of Obstetrics and Gynaecology* **94**, 267−9.
Alexander J.I. & Spence A.A. (1973) Apparent improvement in postoperative lung volumes by using the Entonox apparatus. *British Journal of Anaesthesia* **45**, 90−2.
Alexander J.I., Spence A.A., Parikh R.K. & Stuart B. (1973) The role of airway closure in postoperative hypoxaemia. *British Journal of Anaesthesia* **45**, 34−40.
Ali J., Yaffe C. & Serrette C. (1981) The effect of transcutaneous electrical nerve stimulation on postoperative pain and pulmonary function. *Surgery* **89**, 502−7.
Armitage E.N. (1979) Caudal block in children. *Anaesthesia* **34**, 396.
Asari H., Inove K., Shibata T. & Soga T. (1981) Segmental effect of morphine injected into the epidural space in man. *Anaesthesiology* **54**, 75−7.
Austin K.L., Stapleton J.V. & Mather L.E. (1980) Relationship between blood meperidine concentrations and analgesic response: a preliminary report. *Anesthesiology* **53**, 460−6.
Bahar M., Rosen M. & Vickers M.D. (1985) Self-administered nalbuphine, morphine and pethidine. *Anaesthesia* **40**, 529−32.
Basbaum A.I., Morley N.J.E., O'Keefe J. & Clanton C.H. (1977) Reversal of morphine and stimulus-produced analgesia by subtotal spinal cord lesions. *Pain* **3**, 43−56.
Beaver W.T., Wallenstein S.L., Houde R.W. & Rogers A. (1966) A comparison of the analgesic effects of methotrimeprazine and morphine in patients with cancer. *Clinical pharmacology and Therapeutics* **5**, 436−46.
Beeley L. (1986) Drugs and breast feeding. In *Clinics in Obstetrics and Gynaecology* Vol. 13, No. 2 (eds Stirrat G. & Beeley L.). W.B. Saunders Co., London.
Bentley J.B., Boral J.D., Nenad R.E. & Gillespie T.J. (1982) Age and fentanyl pharmacokinetics. *Anesthesia and Analgesia* **61**, 968−71.
Bowsher D. (1981) A note on the distinction between first and second pain. In *Anatomical, Physiological and Pharmacological Aspects of Trigeminal Pain* (eds Matthews B. & Hill R.G.). Excerpta Medica, Amsterdam.
Boyes R.N., Scott D.B., Jebson P.J., Godman M.J. & Julian D.G. (1971)

Pharmacokinetics of lignocaine in man. *Clinical Pharmacology and Therapeutics* **12**, 105−16.
Brodal A. (1981) *Neurological Anatomy*, 3rd Edition. Oxford University Press, Oxford.
Bromage P.R., Burfoot M.F., Crowell D.E. & Pettigrew R.T. (1964) Quality of epidural blockade. 1. Influence of physical factors. *British Journal of Anaesthesia* **36**, 342−52.
Bromage P.R., Camporesi E. & Chesnut D. (1980) Epidural narcotics for postoperative analgesia. *Anesthesia and Analgesia* **59**, 473−80.
Bromage P., Camporesi E., Durant P. & Nielsen C. (1982) Rostral spread of epidural morphine. *Anesthesiology* **56**, 431−6.
Brownridge P. (1983) Epidural and intrathecal opiates for postoperative pain relief. *Anaesthesia* **38**, 74−5.
Buck S.H. & Burks T.F. (1986) The neuropharmacology of capsaicin: review of some recent observations. *Pharmacological Reviews* **38**, 179−226.
Budd K. (1981) Non-analgesic drugs in the management of pain. In *Persistent Pain, Modern Methods of Treatment* (eds Lipton S. & Miles J.) **3**, 223−40. Academic Press, London.
Bullingham R.E.S., McQuay H.J. & Moore R.A. (1982) Extradural and intrathecal narcotics. In *Recent Advances in Anaesthesia and Analgesia* (eds Atkinson R.S. & Langton-Hewer C.) no. 14. Churchill Livingstone, London.
Bulmer J.N. & Duckett A.C. (1985) Absorption of lignocaine through split skin donor sites. *Anaesthesia* **40**, 808−9.
Bussey J.G. & Jackson A. (1981) TENS for post-surgical analgesia. *Contemporary Surgery* **18**, 35−41.
Caldwell J., Wakile L.A. & Notarriani L.J. (1978) Maternal and neonatal disposition of pethidine in childbirth — a study using quantitative gas chromatography−mass spectrography. *Life Sciences* **22**, 589−96.
Campbell D. (1977) The management of postoperative pain. In *Pain: New Perspectives in Measurements and Management* (eds Marcus A.W., Smith R. & Whittle B.). Churchill Livingstone, Edinburgh.
Chapman C.R. (1985) Psychological factors in postoperative pain. In *Acute Pain* (eds Smith G. & Covino B.G.). Butterworths, London.
Chapman C.R., Wilson M.E. & Gehrig J.D. (1976) Comparative effects of acupuncture and transcutaneous stimulation on the perception of painful dental stimuli. *Pain* **2**, 265−83.
Chapman C.R., Chin A.C.N. & Haskins S.W. (1979) Brain evoked potentials as correlates of laboratory pain: a review and perspective. In *Advances in Pain Research and Therapy* Vol. 3 (ed. Bonica J.J.), 791−803. Raven Press, New York.
Christensen P. & Brandt M.R. (1982) Extradural morphine and Stokes−Adams attacks. *British Journal of Anaesthesia* **54**, 363.
Chrubasik J., Scholler K.L., Wiemers K. & Friedrich G. (1984) Low-dose infusion of morphine prevents respiratory depression. *Lancet* **1**, 793.
Cohen M.R., Pickar D., Dubois M. & Burney W.E. (1982) Stress induced plasma beta-endorphin immunoreactivity may predict postoperative morphine usage. *Psychiatric Research* **6**, 7−12.

References

Cooperman A.M., Hall B., Sadar E.S. & Hardy R.W. (1975) Use of transcutaneous electrical stimulation in the control of postoperative pain. *Surgical Forum* **26**, 77–8.

Corke C.F. & Wheatley R.G. (1985) Respiratory depression complicating epidural diamorphine. Two case reports of administration after dural puncture. *Anaesthesia* **40**, 1203–5.

Corning J.L. (1885) Spinal anaesthesia and local medication of the cord. *New York Medical Journal* **42**, 483–5.

Cousins M. & Bridenbaugh P.O. (1980) *Neural Blockade for Pain and Pain Relief* Philadelphia, J.B. Lippincott Co.

Craig D.B. (1981) Postoperative recovery of pulmonary function. *Anaesthesia and Analgesia* **60**, 46–52.

Cronin K.D. & Davies M.J. (1976) Intercostal block for postoperative pain relief. *Anaesthesia and Intensive Care* **4**, 259–61.

Dalrymple D.G., Parbrook G.D. & Steel D.F. (1973) Factors predisposing to postoperative pain and pulmonary complications. *British Journal of Anaesthesia* **45**, 589–97.

Dodson M.E. (1985) *The Management of Postoperative Pain*. Edward Arnold, London.

Duggan A.W., Hall J.B. & Headley P.M. (1976) Morphine, enkephalin and the substantia gelatinosa. *Nature* **264**, 456–8.

Edelbroek P.M., Linssen A.C.G., Zitman F.G., Rooymans H.G.M, & de Woolf F.A. (1986) Analgesic and antidepressive effects of low-dose amitriptyline in relation to its metabolism in patients. *Clinical Pharmacology and Therapeutics* **39**, 159–62.

Ellis R., Haines D., Shah R., Cotton R. & Smith G. (1982) Pain relief after abdominal surgery — a comparison of i.m. morphine, sublingual buprenorphine and self-administered i.v. pethidine. *British Journal of Anaesthesia* **54**, 421–8.

Engberg G. (1978) Relief of postoperative pain with intercostal blockade compared with the use of narcotic drugs. *Acta Anaesthesiologica Scandinavica*, Suppl. **70**, 36–8.

Engquist A., Jorgensen B.C. & Andersen H.B. (1981) Catatonia after epidural morphine. *Acta Anaesthesiologica Scandinavica* **25**, 445–6.

Fell O., Chemielewski A. & Smith G. (1982) Postoperative analgesia with controlled release morphine sulphate. *British Medical Journal* **285**, 92–4.

Ferreira S.H. (1972) Prostaglandins, aspirin-like drugs and analgesia. *Nature* **240**, 200–3.

Fletcher J.E. (1985) PhD Thesis, University of Bristol.

Forrest W.H., Brown B.W., Brown C.R., Defalque R., Gold M., Gordon H.E., James K.E., Datz J., Mahler D.L., Shroff P. & Teutsch G. (1977) Dextroamphetamine with morphine for the treatment of postoperative pain. *New England Journal of Medicine* **269**, 712–15.

Fournie-Zaluski M.C., Chaillet P., Bouboutou R., Coulaud A., Cherot P., Waksman G., Costentin J. & Roques B.P. (1984) Analgesic effects of kelatorphan, a new highly potent inhibitor of multiple enkephalin-degrading enzymes. *European Journal of Pharmacology* **102**, 525–8.

Gibbs J.M., Johnson H.D. & Davis F.M. (1982) Patient administration of i.v.

References

buprenorphine for postoperative pain relief using the 'Cardiff' demand analgesia apparatus. *British Journal of Anaesthesia* **54**, 279–84.

Goudie T.A., Allen M.W.B., Lonsdale M. *et al.* (1985) Continuous subcutaneous infusion of morphine for postoperative pain. *Anaesthesia* **40**, 1086–92.

Green R. & Dawkins C.J.M. (1966) Postoperative analgesia: the use of a continuous drip epidural block. *Anaesthesia* **21**, 372.

Gullo A. & Romano E. (1983) Naloxone and anaphylactic shock. *Lancet* **1**, 819.

Gustafsson L.L., Ackerman S., Adamson H., Rane A. & Schildt (1982) Disposition of morphine in cerebrospinal fluid after epidural administration. *Lancet* **1**, 796.

Hallin R.G., Torebjork H.E. & Wiesenfeld Z. (1982) Nociceptors and warm receptors innervated by C fibres in human skin. *Journal of Neurology, Neurosurgery and Psychiatry* **45**, 313–19.

Hashemi K. & Middleton M.D. (1983) Subcutaneous bupivacaine for postoperative analgesia after herniorrhaphy. *Annals of the Royal College of Surgeons* **65**, 38–9.

Hayes A.G., Skingle M. & Tyers M.B. (1986) Reversal by β-funaltrexamine of the antinociceptive effect of opioid agonists in the rat. *British Journal of Pharmacology* **88**, 867–72.

Henderson G. (1983) Electrophysiological analysis of opioid action. *British Medical Bulletin* **39**, 59–64.

Henry J. & Volans G. (1984) ABC of poisoning. analgesics: opioids. *British Medical Journal* **289**, 990–3.

Hill R.G., Morris R. & Pepper C.M. (1984) Electrophysiological studies on the actions of opioids with particular reference to the production of analgesia. In *Opioids Past, Present and Future* (eds Hughes J., Collier H.O.J., Rance M.J. & Tyers M.B.), 61–78. Taylor & Francis, London.

Hill H., Gramm H.J. & Link J. (1986) Changes in intracranial pressure associated with extradural anaesthesia. *British Journal of Anaesthesia* **58**, 676–80.

Houde R.W. (1966) On assaying analgesics in man. In *Pain* (eds Knighton R.S. & Dumke P.R.), pp. 183–96. Little, Brown & Co., Boston.

Hughes D.G. (1985) Intra-articular bupivacaine for pain relief in arthroscopic surgery. *Anaesthesia* **40**, 821.

Hughes J. (1983) Opioid peptides. *British Medical Bulletin* **39**, 1–106.

Hymes A.C., Raab D.E., Yonehiro E.G., Nelson G.D. & Printy A.L. (1973) Electrical surface stimulation for control of acute postoperative pain and prevention of ileus. *Surgical Forum* **24**, 447–9.

Hymes A.C., Yonehiro E.G., Raab D.E., Nelson G.D. & Printy A.L. (1974) Electrical stimulation for treatment and prevention of ileus and atelectasis. *Surgical Forum* **25**, 222–4.

Ishizuka E., Iwasaki A. & Kobayashi P. (1979) Continuous intercostal nerve block for pain relief after lumbar incision. *Journal of Urology* **122**, 506–7.

Jack R.D. (1975) Regional anaesthesia for pain relief. *British Journal of Anaesthesia* **47**, 278–80.

Jackson H.C. & Sewell R.D.E. (1986) Characterization of the effects of

(+)meptazinol, its individual enantiomers and N-methylmeptazinol on food consumption in the rat. *British Journal of Pharmacology* **88**, 689–95.

Judkins K.C. & Harmer M. (1982) Haloperidol as an adjunct in the management of postoperative pain. *Anaesthesia* **37**, 1118–20.

Jurna I., Grossman W. & Theres C. (1973) Inhibition by morphine of repetitive activation of cat spinal motoneurones. *Neuropharmacology* **12**, 983–93.

Kakkar V.V., Corrigan T.P. & Fossard D.P. (1975) Prevention of fatal postoperative pulmonary embolism by low doses of heparin. *Lancet* **ii**, 45–51.

Kay B. (1981) Postoperative pain relief. Use of an on-demand analgesia computer (ODAC) and a comparison of the rate of use of fentanyl and alfentanil. *Anaesthesia* **36**, 949–51.

Kirno K. & Lindell K. (1986) Intercostal nerve blockade. *British Journal of Anaesthesia* **58**, 246.

Koehntop D.E., Rodman J.H., Brundage D.M., Hegland M.G. & Buckley J.J. (1986) Pharmacokinetics of fentanyl in neonates. *Anesthesia and Analgesia* **65**, 227–32.

Lasagna L. & Beecher H.K. (1954) The optimal dose of morphine. *Journal of the American Medical Association* **156**, 230–4.

Lawrie B.R., & Drake J. (1985) Delayed cardiorespiratory depression following nalbuphine administration. *Anaesthesia* **40**, 1139–40.

Le Bars D., Guilbaud G., Jurna I. & Besson J.M. (1976) Differential effects of morphine on response of dorsal horn lamina V type cells elicited by A and C fibre stimulation in the spinal cat. *Brain Research* **115**, 518–24.

Lecomte J-M., Costentin J., Vlaiculescu A., Chailet P., Marcais-Collado H., Llorens-Cortes C., LeBoyer M. & Schwartz J-C. (1986) Pharmacological properties of acetorphan, a parenterally active 'enkephalinase' inhibitor. *Journal of Pharmacology and Experimental Therapeutics* **237**, 937–44.

Levine J.D. & Gordon N.C. (1982) Pain in prelingual children and its evaluation by pain induced vocalization. *Pain* **14**, 85–93.

Lewis V.L. & Thompson W.A.L. (1953) Reduction of postoperative pain. *British Medical Journal* **1**, 973–4.

Lockhart A.S, & Francis R.I. (1986) Epidural meptazinol. *Anaesthesia* **41**, 88–9.

Long D.M. & Hagfors N. (1975) Electrical stimulation in the nervous system: current status of electrical stimulation of the nervous system for relief of pain. *Pain* **1**, 109–23.

McQuay H.G. & Moore A. (1984) Metabolism of narcotics. *British Medical Journal* **288**, 237.

Martin W.R., Eades C.G., Thompson J.A., Huppler R.E. & Gilbert P.E. (1976) The effect of morphine- and nalorphine-like drugs in the nondependent and morphine-dependent chronic spinal dog. *Journal of Pharmacology and Experimental Therapeutics* **197**, 517-32.

Mather L.E., Tucker G.T., Pflug A.E., Lindop M.J. & Wilkerson C. (1975) Meperidine kinetics in man. *Clinical Pharmacology and Therapeutics* **17**, 21–30.

Misra A.L., Potani R.B. & Vadlamani N.L. (1987) Sterospecific potentiation of opiate analgesia by cocaine: predominant role of noradrenaline. *Pain* **28**, 129−38.

Moller R.A. & Covino B.G. (1985) Toxic cardiac electrophysiologic effects of bupivacaine and lidocaine at high concentrations. *Anesthesiology* **63**, A223.

Moore R.A. & McQuay H.J. (1985) In *Acute Pain* (eds Smith G. & Covino B.G.), pp. 133−54. Butterworths, London.

Moore R.A., Bullingham R.E.S., McQuay H.J., Hand C.W., Aspel J.B., Allen M.C. & Thomas D. (1982) Dural permeability to narcotics: *in vitro* determination and application to extradural administration. *British Journal of Anaesthesia* **54**, 1117−28.

Moore A., Bullingham R., McQuay H., Allen M., Baldwin D., & Cole A. (1984) Spinal fluid kinetics of morphine and heroin. *Clinical Pharmacology and Therapeutics* **35**, 40−5.

Morris T. & Tracey J. (1977) Lignocaine: its effects on wound healing. *British Journal of Surgery* **64**, 902−03.

Morrison J.D., Loan W.B. & Dundee J.W. (1971) Controlled comparison of the efficacy of fourteen preparations in the relief of postoperative pain. *British Medical Journal* **3**, 287−90.

Muir F.G. (1985) Penile block in awake children. *Anaesthesia* **50**, 1021−2.

Nayman J. (1979) Measurement and control of postoperative pain. *Annals of the Royal College of Surgeons* **61**, 419−29.

Norris W. & Baird W.L.M. (1967) Pre-operative anxiety: a study of its incidence and aetiology. *British Journal of Anaesthesia* **39**, 503−9.

North R.A. & Egan T. (1983) Opioid peptides in peripheral tissues. *British Medical Bulletin* **39**, 71−5.

Nunn J.F. & Slavin G. (1980) Posterior intercostal nerve block for pain relief after cholecystectomy: anatomical basis and efficacy. *British Journal of Anaesthesia* **52**, 253−60.

Owen H. & Galloway P.J. (1984) The effect of incisional infiltration of 0.5% bupivacaine on pain after surgery. *British Journal of Anaesthesia* **56**, 1292−3.

Parbrook G.D. (1966) Postoperative pain relief: comparison of methadone and morphine when used concurrently with nitrous oxide analgesia. *British Medical Journal* **2**, 616−18.

Parbrook G.D., Steel D.F. & Dalrymple, D.G. (1973) Factors predisposing to postoperative pain and pulmonary complications. *British Journal of Anaesthesia* **45** 21−33.

Pasternak G.W. (1980) Multiple opiate receptors: (3H) ethylketocyclazocine receptor binding and ketocyclazocine analgesia. *Proceedings of the National Academy of Sciences of the U.S.A.* **77**, 3691−4.

Petrovsky B.V. & Yefuni S.N. (1965) Therapeutic inhalational anaesthesia. *British Journal of Anaesthesia* **37**, 42.

Pike P.M.H. (1978) Transcutaneous electrical stimulation. *Anaesthesia* **33**, 165−71.

Procacci P., Della Corte M., Zoppi M., Romano S., Maresca M. & Voegelin M.R. (1974) Pain threshold measurements in man. In *Recent Advances on*

Pain (eds Bonica J.J., Procacci P. & Pagni C.A.), 105–47. Thomas, Springfield, Illinois.

Rapeport W.G., Rogers K.M., McCubbin T.D., Agnew E. & Brodie M.J. (1984) Treatment of intractable neurogenic pain with carbamazepine. *Scottish Medical Journal* **29**, 162-5.

Rawal N., Arner A., Gustafsson L.L. & Allvin R. (1987) Present state of intrathecal opioid analgesia in Sweden. A nationwide followup survey. *British Journal of Anaesthesia* **59**, 800–5.

Reiz S. & Westburg M. (1980) Side effects of epidural morphine. *Lancet* **2**, 203–4.

Reiz S., Ahoing J., Ahrenfelt B., Andersson M. & Andersson S. (1981) Epidural morphine for postoperative pain relief. *Acta Anaesthesiologica Scandinavica* **25**, 111–14.

Rigg J.R.A., Browne R.A., Davis C. *et al.* (1978) Variation in the disposition of morphine after intramuscular administration in surgical patients. *British Journal of Anaesthesia* **50**, 1125–30.

Rodriguez R.E., Leighton G., Hill R.G. & Hughes J. (1986) *In vivo* evidence for spinal delta-opiate receptor-operated antinociception. *Neuropeptides* **8**, 221–41.

Rosenblatt R., Papitone-Rockwell R. & McKillop R.J. (1979) Continuous axillary analgesia for traumatic hand injury. *Anaesthesiology* **51**, 565–6.

Samarji W.N. (1977) Rectus sheath analgesia in the control of postoperative abdominal pain and its influence on pulmonary function and pulmonary complications. In *Proceedings of the 5th World congress of Anaesthesiology* (Kyoto). Excerpta Medica, Amsterdam.

Saunders C. (1981) Current views of pain relief in terminal care. In *The Therapy of Pain* (ed. Swerdlow M.), 215–41. MTP Press, Lancaster.

Schmidt J.F., Chraemmer-Jorgensen B., Pedersen J.E. & Risbo A. (1985) Postoperative pain relief with naloxone. Sever respiratory depression and pain after high-dose buprenorphine. *Anaesthesia* **40**, 583–6.

Scott L.E., & Clum G.A. (1984) Examining the interaction effects of coping style and brief intervention in the treatment of postsurgical pain. *Pain* **20**, 279–92.

Sechzer P.H. (1968) Objective measurement of pain. *Anesthesiology* **29**, 209–10.

Sheehan, M.J., Hayes A.G. & Tyers M.B. (1986) Pharmacology of δ-opioid receptors in the hamster vas deferens. *European Journal of Pharmacology* **130**, 57–64.

Simpson P.J. Hughes D.J. & Long D.M. (1982) Prolonged local anaesthesia for inguinal herniorrhaphy with bupivacaine and dextran. *Annals of the Royal College of Surgeons of England* **64**, 243–6.

Smith T.W., Buchan P., Parsons D.N. & Wilkinson (1982) Peripheral antinociceptive effects of *N*-methylmorphine. *Life Sciences* **31**, 1205–8

Solomon R.A., Viernstein M.C. & Long D.M. (1980) Reduction of postoperative pain and narcotic use by transcutaneous electrical nerve stimulation. *Surgery* **87**, 142–6.

Spence A.A. & Smith G. (1971) Postoperative analgesia and lung function: a comparision of morphine with extradural block. *British Journal of Anaesthesia* **43**, 144–8.

Stanski D.R., Greenblatt D.J. & Lowenstein E. (1978) Kinetics of intravenous and intramuscular morphine. *Clinical Pharmacology and Therapeutics* **24**, 52–9.

Streltze J. & Wade T.C. (1981) The influence of cultural group on the undertreatment of postoperative pain. *Psychosomatic Medicine* **43**, 397–403.

Sung Y.F., Kutner M.H., Cerine F.C. & Frederickson E.L. (1977) Comparison of the effects of acupuncture and codeine on postoperative dental pain. *Anesthesia and Analgesia: Current Researches* **56**, 473–8.

Swerdlow M. & Jones R. (1970) The duration of action of bupivicaine, prilocaine and lignocaine. *British Journal of Anaesthesia* **42**, 335–9.

Thomas D.F.M., Lambert W.G. & Williams K.L. (1983) The direct perfusion of surgical wounds with local anaesthetic solution: an approach to postoperative pain. *Annals of the Royal College of Surgeons* **65**, 226.

Thomas T.A., & Griffiths M.J. (1982) A pain slide rule. *Anaesthesia* **37**, 960–1.

Thomas T.A., Fletcher J.E. & Hill R.G. (1982) Influence of medication, pain and progress in labour on plasma β-endorphin-like immunoreactivity. *British Journal of Anaesthesia* **54**, 401–8.

Twycross R.G. (1979) The effect of cocaine in the Brompton cocktail. *Advances in Pain research and therapy* **3**, 927–32.

Tyers M.B., Hayes A.G. & Sheehan M.J. (1986) The animal pharmacology of novel opioid analgesic drug, xorphanol. *NIDA Monograph Series* **75**, 698.

Wall P.D. (1984) Mechanisms of acute and chronic pain. In *Advances in Pain Research and Therapy. Vol.6, Neural Mechanisms of Pain* (eds Lawrence K. & Liebeskind J.), 95–104. Raven Press, New York.

Watson J., Moore A., McQuay H., Teddy P., Baldwin D., Allen N., & Bullingham R. (1984) Plasma morphine concentrations and analgesic effects of lumbar extradural morphine and heroin. *Anesthesia and Analgesia* **63**, 629–34.

Way W.L., Costley E.C, & Way E.L.I. (1965) Respiratory sensitivity of the new-born infant to meperidine and morphine. *Clinical Pharmacology and Therapeutics* **6**, 454–61.

Welchew E.A. (1982) A postoperative pain recorder: a patient-controlled device for assessing postoperative pain. *Anaesthesia* **37**, 838–41.

White J.B., & Stow P. (1985) Rationale and experience with visual analogue toys. *Anaesthesia* **40**, 601–3.

Wikler A. (1950) Sites and mechanisms of action of morphine and related drugs in the central nervous system. *Pharmacological Reviews* **2**, 435–506.

Williams J.T., Egan T.M. & North R.A. (1982) Enkephalin opens potassium channels on mammalian central neurones. *Nature* **299**, 74–7.

Woodrow K.M., Friedman D.G., Siegelaub A.B. *et al.* (1972) Pain tolerance: differences according to age, sex and race. *Psychosomatic Medicine* **34**, 548–56.

Yaksh T.L. (1981) Spinal opiate analgesia: characteristics and principles of action. *Pain* **11**, 293–346.

Yaksh T.L., Jessell T.M., Gamse R., Mudge A. & Leeman S. (1980) Intrathecal morphine inhibits substance P release from mammalian spinal cord *in vivo*. *Nature* **286**, 155–7.

Yaksh T.L. Atchinson S.R. & Durant P.A.C. (1986) Characteristics of action and pharmacology of intrathecally administered DALA^2–DLEU^5 enkephalin. *Advances in Pain Research and Therapy* **8**, 303–14.

Further Reading

Bond M.R. (1980) Personality and pain: the influence of psychological and environmental factors upon the experience of pain in hospital patients. In *Persistent Pain* Vol. 2 (ed. Lipton S.), pp. 1–25. Grune & Stratton, New York.

Bullingham R.E.S. (ed.) (1983) *Clinics in Anaesthesiology — Opiate Analgesia*. 236 pp. W.B. Saunders, London.

Cousins M. & Bridenbaugh P.O. (eds) (1980) *Neural Blockade in Clinical Anaesthesia and Management of Pain*, 749 pp. J.B. Lippincott Co., Philadelphia.

Cousins M. & Phillips G. (eds) (1986) *Acute Pain Management*. 300 pp. Churchill Livingstone, Edinburgh.

Covino B. & Vassallo H. (1976) *Local Anesthetics: Mechanisms of Action and Clinical Use*. 173 pp. Grune & Stratton, New York.

Davies D.M. (ed.) *Textbook of Adverse Drug Reactions*, 2nd Edition. 680 pp. Oxford University Press, Oxford.

Dodson M. (1985) *The Management of Postoperative Pain*. 274 pp. Edward Arnold, London.

Goodman Gilman A., Goodman L., Rall T. & Murad F. (eds) (1985) *Goodman & Gilman's The Pharmacological Basis of Therapeutics*, 7th Edition. 1843 pp. Macmillan Publishing Company, New York.

Harmer M., Rosen M. & Vickers M.D. (eds) (1985) *Patient-Controlled Analgesia*. 216 pp. Blackwell Scientific Publications, Oxford.

Hosking J. & Welchew E. (1985) *Postoperative Pain: Understanding its Nature and How to Treat It*. 175 pp. Faber & Faber, London.

Kruger L. & Liebeskind J. (eds) (1984) *Advances in Pain Research and Therapy*: Vol. 6, *Neural Mechanisms of Pain*. 364 pp. Raven Press, New York.

Lewis T. (1942) *Pain*. 192 pp. (facsimile edition 1981). The MacMillan Press, London.

Marcus A.W., Smith R. & Whittle B. (eds) (1977) *Pain—New Perspectives in Measurement and Management*. 194pp. Churchill Livingstone, Edinburgh.

Prys-Roberts C. & Hug C.C. Jr (1984) *Pharmacokinetics of Anaesthesia*. 368 pp. Blackwell Scientific Publications, Oxford.

Rizzi R. & Visetin M. (eds) (1984) *Pain — Proceedings of Joint Meeting of the European Chapters of the International Association for the Study of Pain*. 488 pp. Piccin/Butterworths, Padua/London.

Smith G. & Covino B. (eds) (1985) *Acute Pain*. 283 pp. Butterworths, London.

Sofaer B. (1984) *Pain: a Handbook for Nurses*. 86 pp. Harper & Row, London.
Wall P.D. & Melsack R. (eds) (1985) *Textbook of Pain*. 866 pp. Churchill Livingstone, Edinburgh.

Index

Aβ fibres 21, 25
Aδ fibres 21–25, 27
Abdominal operation, site of epidural puncture with 166
Abdominal wall spasm 48, 195–6
Absorption 198–201
  abnormal, overdosage rsulting from 238
  drug interactions affecting 219–23, 232, 234,
  proportion and rate 119, 152
  reduction 239–40
Acetaminophen *see* Paracetamol
Acetorphan, pharmacology 94
Acetylcysteine, paracetamol overdose treated with 244
Acid–base balance, effects on drug distribution and elimination 215–16
Activity of sensory neurones, recording 22
Acupuncture 127
Acute *v.* chronic pain 245–6
Addiction, drug, problems presented by 43–5
Administration of anaesthesia and analgesia. *See under* Anaesthetics, local/regional; Analgesic drugs
Admission, hospital, reducing stress of 40–1
Adrenaline, postoperative levels 52
Adrenergic drugs, action 54, 87, 229
Adrenocorticotrophic hormone, postoperative levels 51
Affect of pain, assessment 7
Afferent input, neuronal response to, depression 69–70
Afferent transmitter release, prevention 69
Age (of patient)
  drug distribution and elimination related to 186, 188, 196, 212–13

opioid side-effects related to 179, 186–7, 197
pain severity and 35–6
Aged, pain relief for 196–7
Agonists
  alpha$_2$ receptor 87–8
  definition 231
  opioid 57, 66–79
    choice 134–8
    full 65–75
    partial 65, 76, 80, 134–5
    pharmacological actions 62
    receptor selectivity 63
Alfentanil
  pharmacokinetics 207
  pharmacology 74
Algogens 27, 28, 88
Allergic reactions to anaesthetics/analgesics 151–2, 187
Alpha$_2$ receptor agonists, pharmacology 87–8
Amino acid transmitters (excitatory amino acids) 30, 86 *See also specific amino acid*
Amphetamine, pharmacology 90–1
Anaesthetics (and anaesthesia)
  drug distribution and elimination affected by 214
  local/regional *See* Anaesthetics, local/regional
  recovery from, explaining to patient about 41–2
Anaesthetics, local/regional (and local analgesia)
  actions (s)
    prolongation, methods for 97, 154
    sites and mechanisms 95–6
    unwanted 96, 118, 145–52
  administration (=anaesthesia) 156–68
    feasibility, site of pain determining 114
    procedural requirements 158–9

260

Index

systemic analgesia compared with 117–18
techniques 156–74
advantages 118, 141, 142–3
choice 152–3
complications and their avoidance 145–52
concentration 164–5
contraindications 144–5
for day-cases, problems 192–4
disadvantages 96, 118, 141–2, 143–4, 155, 157–60
distribution and elimination, factors affecting 215–16, 221–3
drugs interacting with 235–7
equipment 158–9
future requirements 229
new 99
opioid plus, combinations 138–9
side-effects 96, 118–19
spread 165–6
volume 164–5
Analgesic corridor 123, 124
Analgesic drugs
administration (=analgesia) 114–27, 135–8, 153–74, 184
improved, costs 19
local *See* Anaesthetics, local/regional (and local analgesia)
methods 114–27, 152–74, 184
patient-controlled 13, 116, 124–7
routes *See* Routes of analgesic administration
supervision 101–3
choice 128–39
conditions affecting 106–13
dangers 5, 145, 148–52, 240–4
new 79–81, 99, 229–30
pharmacology 56–99
secondary 89–94
systemically administered 117–18, 117–24
choice 128–39
future requirements 229–30
trials, assessment of 16–19
Analogue scale, visual 8–12
Antagonist(s)
bradykinin 88
definition/mechanism of actions 231, 232
opioid 57, 65, 66, 76–9, 241

choice 134–5
Anterior pituitary hormones, postoperative levels 50–1
Anticonvulsants, analgesic 89
Antidepressants, analgesic 90
Antidiuretic hormone (8-arginine vasopressin), postoperative levels 53–4
Anti-inflammatory drugs *See* Non-steroidal anti-inflammatory drugs
Antipsychotics with analgesic properties 92
Anxiety, fear and distress 38–9
analgesic choices with 107–8
avoidance measures 40–2
drug distribution and elimination affected by 214
with local anaesthesia 148–9
Arachidonic acid metabolism 82, 83
Aspirin (and other salicylates)
in breast milk 195
distribution and elimination, pH effects 216
toxicity in neonates/infants 187, 195
Assessment of pain 6–16 *See also* Measurement
Asthma, analgesic choices with 84, 107
Atopy 151–2, 187
Attendants *See* Staff
Autologous blood patches 163–4
Automatic (and semi-automatic) systems of measuring pain severity 10–11
Autonomic changes with acute and chronic pain 245
Availability, bio-, of drugs 201–2

Babies, pain relief 185–9
Baclofen, pharmacology 94
Benzodiazepines, pharmacology 92
Biliary duct spasm 195
Binding, receptor *See* Receptors *and specific (types of) receptors*
Bioavailability of drugs 201–2
Biochemical tests, pain assessment using 16

Biotransformation of analgesics
    207–9, 211, 217–18
  drug interactions affecting 219,
    222, 235, 236
Bleeding with local anaesthetics 147
Blood
  gases
    effects of pain on 49
    pain severity measured from 15
  levels of drugs, maintaining
    constant 204–6
Brachial plexus cannulation,
    equipment for 159
Bradycardia risks with local
    anaesthesics 148
Bradykinin antagonists,
    pharmacology 88
Brain
  cortex 26–7
  opioid receptors in 62
  stem 26, 27, 31
Breast feeding, analgesia and 194–5
Breathing *See* Ventilation and
    respiration
Bremazocine 79, 80
  spinally applied 182
Bronchospasm 84, 107, 152
Bupivacaine 98, 152–3
Buprenorphine 137
  overdosage, management 241
  pharmacology 76
  spinally applied 181, 183
Butorphanol, pharmacology 78
Butyrophenones, pharmacology, 92

C fibres 21, 22, 23, 24, 25
Cannulation 154–6, 160
  equipment 158–9
  future requirements 225–6
Capsaicin 99, 100, 229
Carbamazepine
  efects on microsomal enzyme
    system 218
  pharmacology 89
Carbon dioxide levels, effects of pain
    on 49
Cardiff Palliator 125
Cardiovascular actions/diseases etc.
    See Heart

Care of patient, psychological aspects
    40–2
Catheter
  intercostal 169
  tip, site, in epidural puncture
    166–7
Caudal blocks in children 171
Causalgia (sympathetic dystrophy)
    35, 245–6
Central nervous system,
    neurotransmitters within
    29–31
Cephalad spread of opioids within
    CSF 176–8, 179
Cerebral cortex 26–7
Cerebrospinal fluid
  distribution and levels of opioids
    in 16, 175–8, 179
  loss 163
Character of pain *See* Quality of
    pain
Chemical messengers 27 *See also*
    Neurotransmitters
Chest, postoperative (syndrome) 47
Children
  caudal blocks in 171
  pain relicf 185–9
  pain scores for 11
  psychological stress in reducing 40
Chloroprocaine 98, 153
Choices in postoperative pain
    management 101–40
  local anaesthesia 152–3, 164–7
Chronic *v*. acute pain relief 245–6
Cimetidine, effects on liver
    function 218, 221, 232
Clearance *See* Elimination;
    Excretion
Clonidine 44, 87–8, 137, 229
Clotting factors, reduced levels.
    analgesic choice with 106,
    145
Cocaine
  in anaesthesia 97
  pharmacology 91, 97
Codeine, pharmacology 72–3
  use 191
Coeliac plexus block, equipment
    for 159
Combinations, drug 138–9
Complaints of pain by patient
  frequency of, significance 4
  psychological factors affecting
    37–8

Index

Complications
  of local anaesthesia 145−52
    avoiding 152
  of pain 46−55
Concentration (of drugs)
  absorption related to 199
  CSF, cord 175
  plasma and tissue 203−4, 205−7
Consciousness, recovery, explaining
    to patient about 41−2
Conditions, analgesics used with
    various 106−13
Consequences of pain 46−55
Continuous analgesia 122−4
  advantages and disadvantages 115
Contraindications for local
    anaesthesia 144−5
Convulsions See under Muscles
Cortex, cerebral 26−7
Cortisol, postoperative levels 52−3
Costs/prices
  of improved analgesia 19, 225
  of pain 1
Cranial injury and surgery, analgesia
    with 109, 190−1
Cryothermy (cryoanalgesia) 174
  for day cases 194
Cultural factors affecting pain
    severity 36
Cyclo-oxygenase inhibitors
  centrally acting 84−5
  opioid plus, combinations 138
  pharmacology 82−5

Damage, tissue, pain caused by,
    mechanism 28−9
Dangers of analgesics 5
Dantrolene, pharmacology 94
Day-case surgery, analgesia 191−4
Definition of pain 1
Delta agonists 81
Delta receptors 62, 63
Demand/requests for analgesics by
    patient 5, 38, 102
  administering analgesics on 122
  advantages and disadvantages 115
Deniers of fear 39
Dependency, drug, problems
    presented by 43−5
Depression of neuronal response to
    afferent input 69−70

Descending inhibitory system, opioid-
    stimulated 69
Description of pain See Words for
    pain
Dextromoramide, pharmacology 75
Dextropropoxyphene, pharmacology
    75
Dezocine, pharmacology 78−9
Diabetes mellitus, analgesic choices
    with 108
Diagnosis, recognition
  of cause of pain 115
  of local anaesthetic toxicity
    150−1
  of overdosage 240−1, 242−3, 244
Diamorphine
  pharmacology, 72, 137
  spinally applied opioids 177, 182
Diclofenac, choice, factors affecting
    132
Differential pain scores 13−14
Diflunisal, choice, factors affecting
    132
Dihydromorphine, pharmacology
    72
Diphenylhydantoin See phenytoin
Dipipanone, pharmacology 75
Disabilities, analgesics used with
    various 106−13
Diseases, analgesics used with
    various, 106−13
Distress See Anxiety
Distribution of drugs 203−5 See
    also Spread
  abnormal 238
  drug interactions affecting 219,
    221
  other factors affecting 212−18
  volume of 203−5, 211
    in the elderly 196
Doctors, analgesia administration and
    the role of 104−5 See also
    Staff
Dorsal horn of spinal cord See
    Spinal cord
Dose
  blood levels related to 205
  local anaesthetics 164−5, 171
  non-steroidal anti-inflammatory
    drugs 132−3
  opioids 136, 137
  over- See Overdose
  size 212
  spinally applied opioids 181−3

Drugs *See also* Anaesthetics;
    Analgesics *and types/names of*
    drugs
  combinations 138−9
  dependence and abuse, problems
    presented by 43−5
  future requirements 229−30
  new 79−81, 99
Duration of action of spinally applied
    opioids 182−3
Dynorphin 57, 58, 59
  pro- 58, 60, 61

Effects of pain 46−55
Elderly, pain relief for 196−7
Electroanaesthesia/electroanalgesia
    228
Electroencephalography
  assessment of hypnosis 228
  pain assessment using 16
Elimination/clearance 205, 207−9
    See also Excretion
  drug interactions affecting 232−3
  other factors affecting 212−18
  time of 211
Embolisms, pulmonary 47, 248
Emotionality, pain severity and
    37−8
Endocrine complications of pain
    50−4
Endoplasmic reticulum,
    biotransformation in
    the 209−10
Endorphin(s) 57, 58, 59
Endorphin-like immunoreactivity 59
  level
    nitrous oxide increasing 85
    measurement 16
  role 59
Enkephalins 57, 58, 59
  breakdown, prevention 93−4
  pro- 58, 60, 61
Entonox demand analgesia 124−5
Enzyme competitors/inhibitors
    93−4, 222
Epidural cannulation 154−5
  equipment 158
  future requirements 225−6
Epidural nerve block/anaesthesia
    157−67
  advantages 160
  anatomy relevant to 160−1

  disadvantages 160
  in the elderly 197
Epidural opioids 175−84
  injection 178
  side-effects 178−81
  spread 178, 182, 184
Epidural puncture
  site, with spinally applied opioids
    183−4
  thoracic 161−2
Epidural space, location, methods
    and devices for 158, 161−3
Epidurography 167
Epinephrine *See* Adrenaline
Equipment
  future requirements 225
  for local anaesthesia 158−9,
    225−6
Ethylketocyclazocine 79, 80
Etidocaine in anaesthesia 98, 153
Excretion 210−11 *See also*
    Elimination
  drug interactions affecting 219,
    222
Expectation by patient of pain relief,
    poor 38
Extradural *See* Epidural
Extroversion and pain perception 37

Fainting with local anaesthesia
    148−9
Fast pain, slow pain and, differences
    between 23
Fatigue (patient), avoidance 42−3
Fear *See* Anxiety
Fenbufen, choice, factors
    affecting 132
Fenoprofen, choice, factors
    affecting 132
Fentanyl
  in neonates and infants 188
  pharmacokinetics 204, 207, 208
    217
  pharmacology 70, 74−5, 137−8
  structure 70
First pain and second pain,
    differences between 23
Fluid balance
  abnormal, analgesics used with
    106
  effect of pain on 53−4
Flupirtine, pharmacology 88

Index

Flurbiprofen, choice, factors affecting 132
Functional residual capacity, pain severity assessed from 15
Future developments in pain relief 225–30

GABA (gamma aminobutyric acid) action 89, 93, 94
Gender *See* Sex
Glucagon, postoperative levels 52, 53
Glucuronide conjugation 209, 212–13
Glutamic acid and neurotransmission 30
Grafts, skin, anaesthesia with 171–2

Haemorrhage with local anaesthesia 147
Headache with epidural anaesthesia, relief 163–4
Head injury/surgery, analgesia with 109, 190–1
Heart
  anaesthetics toxic to 148, 150, 151
  diseases, analgesic choices with 111
  drugs acting on 86, 148, 151
  pain associated with 34
Helplessness, patient's feeling of effects 39
Hepatic conditions/damage etc. *See* Liver
Heroin *See* Diamorphine
Hormones
  effect of pain on 50–4
  interactions 53
Hospital admission, reducing stress of 40–1
Hydrolysis of drugs 209
Hydromorphone, pharmacology 73
5-Hydroxytryptamine 90, 93
5-Hydroxytryptamine receptor agonists 91
5-Hydroxytryptophan 93
Hypersensitivity to anaesthetics/analgesics 151–2, 187
Hypertension, analgesic choices with 109

Hyperthyroidism, analgesic choices with 109
Hypnosis 228
Hypovalaemia/hypovalaemic shock, analgesic choices with 110
Hypoxaemia 48–9
  in the elderly 197

Ibuprofen, choice, factors affecting 132
Iliac crest block 170
Illegal drugs, problems associated with 43–5
Illnesses, analgesics used in various 106–13
Incision, site of, pain severity and the 33 *See also* Wound, operative
Indirect measurements of pain severity 14–16
Indomethacin, choice, factors affecting 132–3
Infants and neonates
  analgesia and breast feeding 194–5
  biotransformation in 207, 209
  pain relief 185–9
Infection
  analgesic choices with 110
  with local anaesthetics 147
Inflammation, pain caused by, mechanism 28–9
Infusion 155, 179, 184
  advantages and disadvantages 155
Injection
  epidural anaesthetics 163
  risks associated with 146–9
Inhalational analgesics, choice, factors affecting 130 *See also* Nasal administration of analgesics
Insulin postoperative levels 51
Intensity of pain *See* Severity of pain
Interactions of drugs 231–7
Intercostal nerve blockade 168–9
Intermittent administration of analgesics *See under* Demand/requests
Intracranial pressure changes, with local anaesthesia 149

raised, analgesia with the possibility of 190–1
Intramuscular administration of analgesics 119, 120
  absorption following 201
Intrathecal opioids 137, 183
Intravenous administration of analgesics 119, 120
  absorption following 200–1
  blood/plasma levels following 203, 205–6
  patient-controlled 125–7
  tissue levels following 206
Isolated arm technique 42
Itch *see* Pruritis

Kappa opioid agonists/analgesics 79–81, 81
  advantages, and disadvantages 81
  overdosage, management 241
Kappa receptors 62, 63
Kelatorphan, pharmacology 93–4
Ketamine
  choice, factors affecting 131, 139
  drugs interacting with 237
  opioid plus, combination 139
  pharmacology 85–6, 87
Ketorolac, pain relief with 84
Kidney
  disease, analgesic choices with 106–7
  excretion 210–11
    effects on drug distribution and elimination 216–17, 219, 222–3
King's Pain Recorder 11

Labour pain, anaesthesia in *See* Obstetric analgesia
Lamina I neurones 24, 25, 26
Lamina II neurones 24, 25
Lamina V neurones 24–5, 26
Levorphanol, pharmacology 73
Lidocaine *See* Lignocaine
Ligand, definition 247
Lignocaine in anaesthesia 97, 153
Lipid-soluble drugs 164, 167–8
  distribution and elimination 177, 204, 216
  opioids 137–8, 175, 177–8, 182

Liver
  biotransformation in the 208–10, 217–8
  conditions, analgesic choices with 106
  damage, paracetamol-associated 243, 244
  functions, effects on drug distribution and elimination 212, 213
Local anaesthesia and analgesia *See* Anaesthetics, local, regional (and local analgesia)
Local complications of local anaesthetics 145–9
Location of pain/operation etc. *See* Site
Lofentanil 138
  spinally applied 181, 183
Lumbar sympathetic block, equipment for 159
Lung
  analgesics administered via 119, 121, 124–5
    absorption 201
  damage, with local anaesthesia 148
  disease, analgesic choices with 111
  embolus 47
  postoperative complications 47–9
  volume/capacity, pain severity measured from 15

McGill pain questionnaire 14
Management *See also* Anaesthetics; Analgesics; Relief, pain
  overdosage 239–40, 241–2, 243, 244
  of pain (postoperative) 101–97
    choices 101–40
    developments 1–2
    nerve blockade for 153–74
    in problem patients 187–9, 189–90, 191, 192–4, 197
  of side-effects/toxicity 151, 181
  surgical/operative, pain worsened by 34
Manpower *See* Staff
Matching of pre-existing and induced pain, pain severity measured via 11

Measurements of pain
  severity 8–16, 19 *See also* Assessment
Mechanisms of pain and pain relief 21–31
Mefenamic acid, choice, factors affecting 133
Membranes, drug passage across 198–9
Memory of pain 5–6
Mental factors affecting pain severity 37–45
Meperidine *See* Pethidine
Meptazinol
  pharmacology 78
  in problem patients 191
Metabolism
  drug 198–224
  in the elderly 197
  effects of pain on 50–3
Metabolites of analgesics 207–10
Methadone
  pharmacology 75
  uses 44, 75
Methionine, paracetamol overdose treated with 244
Methods of administering analgesia 114–27, 153–74, 184
Microsomes
  biotransformation in the 209–10
  enzyme systems of, drugs affecting 218
Milk, breast, analgesics in 194–5
Mineralocorticoids
  activity 54
  deficiency, effects 54
N-Methyl-D-aspartate receptor 86
Modulation of pain perception, role of neurotransmitters in 27
Monitoring
  of analgesic actions 101–2
  respiration *See* Ventilation and respiration
Monoamine (s) 31
Monoamine oxidase inhibitors, pharmacology 90
Monoamine uptake blockers, pharmacology 90
Morphine
  alternatives to 72–81
  bioavailability 202
  distribution and elimination, factors affecting 217
  effects 66–71
    on ADH levels 53
    cocaine-potentiated 91
    in neonates/infants 187–8
  pharmacokinetics 202, 207
  spinally applied 181, 183
  spread 177
  structure 70
Motor blockade 167–8
Mu (-selective) opioid agonists 71
  side-effects 79
Mu receptors 62, 63
  types 64
Muscle
  paralysis, deliberate 167–8
  spasm/convulsions and guarding
    abdominal wall 48, 195–6
    local anaesthetics causing 151
    management 113, 114, 116, 151, 195–6
Myocardial infarction, analgesic choices with 111

Nalbuphine, pharmacology 77
Naloxone 66
  opioid overdosage treated with 241
Naproxen, choice, factors affecting 133
Narcosis in the elderly 197
Narcotic dependence and abuse, problems, presented by 43–5
Nasal administration of analgesics 119, 121 *See also* Inhalational analgesics
NE-19550 99, 100
Needles for local anaesthesia
  future requirements 226
  insertion
    for epidural nerve block 158, 159, 161
    for nerve block 169, 170, 171, 172
  risks associated with 146, 147, 148
Nefopam
  choice, factors affecting 131
  drugs interacting with 237
  pharmacology 87
Neonates *See* Infants and neonates

Nerve
  blockade   143, 153–73, 192–4
    in day-case surgery, problems associated with   192–4
    postoperative   143, 153–74
  damage with local anaesthesia   146, 152
  fibres
    local anaesthesia   95–6, 145, 152
    sensory   21–6
  sheath, cannulation   154–6
  stimulators, future requirements   226
Neurolysis, reversible   174
Neuronal response to afferent input, depression   69–70
Neurone, sensory   21–6
Neurotransmission   29–31
  excitatory   29–30
  inhibitory   30–1
Neurotransmitters   29–31
  modulation of pain perception and   27
  precursors, pharmacology   93–4
  primary afferent, release, prevention   69
Newborn   See Infants and neonates
New drugs
  anaesthetics   99
  analgesics   79–81
Nitrous oxide
  administration   124–5
  analgesic properties   85
  choice, factors affecting   130
Non-opioid analgesics   82–94
  choice   128–31, 138
    versus opioids   128
Non-steroidal anti-inflammatory drugs
  choice, factors affecting   106–13, 114, 129–34, 138
  definition   247
  drugs interacting with   234–5
  opioid plus, combinations   138
  overdosage   242–3
    acute v. chronic   242
  pharmacokinetics   208, 216
  pharmacology   83–4
  in problem patients   191
  trials, assessment in   17
Noradrenaline   29
Norepinephrine   See Noradrenaline
Nurses, analgesia administration and the roles of   104   See also Staff

Obese patients   189–90
  drug distribution and elimination in   213–14
  pain management   189–90
  problems presented by   189
Objective measurements of pain severity   14–16
Obstetric analgesia   183
  site of epidural puncture   166
On-demand analgesic computer   126
  See also Demand/request
Operation
  drug distribution and elimination affected by   214
  pain worsened by   34–5
  site of   See Site
Operative management, pain arising from   34
Opioids   56–81, 134–8, 175–84
  choice   129, 134–9, 181–3
    v. non-opioids   128
  drugs interacting with   232–4
  endogenous   57–61
    measurement   16
    role   31, 66–71
  overdosage   240–2
  pharmacokinetics   207–11, 212–18
    factors affecting   215, 217–18
  pharmacology   56–81
  precursors, structure   58
  in problem patients   187–92, 195–7
  receptors   See Receptors
  spinally applied opioids   137–8, 175–84
  systemic and spinal, concomitant use   179
  withdrawal problems   43–5
Oral administration (of analgesics)   117, 119, 120
  absorption following   199–200
  of opioids   135
Organs   See Tissues, organs and other structures
Origin of pain   See Site
Overdose   149–51, 238–44
  cause   238–9

Index

management 151, 239–40, 241–2, 243, 244
Overweight patients *See* Obese patients
Oxidative reactions, microsomal 209–10
Oxycodone, pharmacology 73
Oxygenation of tissues, maintaining 151
Oxymorphone, pharmacology 73

Pain relief, *see* Relief, pain
Palliator, Cardiff 125
Papaveretum
  in neonates and infants 188
  pharmacology 72
Paravertebral nerve block 173
Paracetamol
  choice, factors affecting 130
  overdosage 243–4
  pharmacology 84
Paralysis, muscle, deliberate 167–8
Pathways of pain and pain relief 21–31
Patient(s)
  demand for analgesics *See* Demands/requests
  involvement in pain relief 13, 103, 105, 116
  memory of pain by 5–6
  problem, pain relief for 185–97
  severity of pain *See* Severity of pain
  view of pain by 3–4
Patient-controlled analgesia 13, 116, 124, 125–7
PCP receptor *See* Sigma receptor
Penile blocks 171
Pentazocine
  pharmacology 76
  spinally applied 182, 183
Peptides as chemical messengers 28, 30, 31
Perception, pain
  factors affecting 35–45
  in neonates and infants, evidence 185–6
  physiological mechanism 23–31
Peripheral nerve block, spinal *v.* 156–7
Personality and pain severity 37–8
Personnel *See* Staff
Pethidine
  dose size 211
  pharmacokinetics 207, 209, 222
  pharmacology 73–4
  spinally applied 181
pH effect on drug distribution and elimination 215–16
Phantom limb pain, management 114
Pharmacodynamics
  definition 247
  drug interactions affecting 232–7
Pharmacokinetics 198–224
  definition 247
  drug interactions affecting 231–7
Pharmacology
  of local anaesthetics 95–100
  of analgesics 56–94
    non-opioid 82–8
    opioid 56–81
    secondary 89–94
Phenazocine, pharmacology 73
Phenothiazines, pharmacology 92
Phenytoin 89
Physical factors affecting pain severity 32–6, 185–90
Physiotherapist, role 42
Piroxicam, choice, factors affecting 122, 133
Pituitary hormones, anterior, postoperative levels 50–1
Placebo effect 18
Plasma levels of drugs 203, 204, 205, 206 *See also* Protein binding
Pneumothorax 48, 49
  risks of, with local anaesthesia 148
Postoperative chest syndrome 47
Postoperative pain relief *See under* Management
Postoperative recovery *See* Recovery
Potency 231
Pregnancy, analgesic choices in 112 *See also* Obstetric anaesthesia
Preoperative patient anxiety 38–9
Preparation for surgery, psychological 40–2
Prices *See* Costs
Prilocaine 98
p.r.n. prescription 102, 248
Problem patients, pain relief for 185–97
Prolactin, postoperative levels 50

Pro-opiomelanocortin 58, 60, 61
Propoxyphene *See*
  Dextropropoxyphene
Prostaglandins, pain enhanced
  by 82–3
Prostanoids
  action 28
  production 82
  role in pain perception process 84
Prostatic hypertrophy, analgesic
  choices with 112
Protein binding (of drugs) 149, 199,
  218, 221
  drug interactions affecting 221,
  234–5, 236
Pruritis 180
Pseudounipolar fibre 21, 28
Psoas sheath block 173
Psychological actions, drugs
  with 90–3
Psychological factors affecting pain
  severity 37–45
Pulmonary function/complications
  etc. *See* Lung

Quality (character) of pain 113–14,
  163
  assessment 6, 7

Racial factors affecting pain severity
  36
Receptors 199, 204, 231–2
  alpha$_2$ 87
  bradykinin 88
  GABA 92–3
  5-hydroxytryptamine 91
  N-methyl-D-aspartate 86
  non-opioid 86, 87, 88
  opioid 61–6, 135
    subtypes 64–5
    types 62–4
Recognition *See* Diagnosis
Recovery, postoperative
  psychological aspects 41–2
  rooms, future requirements 227
Rectal administration (of analgesics)
  119, 121
  absorption following 200
  opioids 135–6
Referred pain, phenomenon of,
  explanation 26, 34

Regular analgesia, advantage and
  disadvantages 115
Relief, pain *See also* Anaesthetics;
  Analgesic drugs; Drugs
  measurement 10
  methods of *See* Management
  physiological mechanisms 21–31
Renal disease, excretion etc. *See*
  Kidney
Requests *See* Demands/requests
Respiration *See* Ventilation and
  respiration
Resuscitation
  with drugs 158, 240–4
  equipment 158, 240–4
Reversible neurolysis 174
Reye syndrome 187
Routes of analgesic administration
  119–21
  choice, considerations 205
  inappropriate, overdosage resulting
    from 149, 238

Salicylates *See* Aspirin
Scale of pain relief, measurement
  10, 13
Scores, pain 8–14, 18–19
  for children 11
  differential 13–14
Second pain, first pain and,
  differences between 23
Sensory decision theory 14
Sensory nerve fibres/neurones 21–6
Serotonin *See*
  5-Hydroxytryptamine
Severity (intensity) of pain 8–16,
  32–45, 103, 114
  factors affecting 32–45
    physical 32–6
    psychological 37–45
  measurement 8–16
Sex hormones, postoperative levels
  51
Sex of patient
  drug distribution and elimination
    related to 213
  pain severity and 36
Sexual organs, pain in region of,
  difficulties in complaining
  of 38
Sharp pain, relief 113
Side-effects/toxicity *See also*
  Overdosage

Index

in children 186–7
of drug metabolites 207–8
in the elderly 197
local anaesthetics 96, 118, 148–52
spinally applied opioids 178–81
systemic analgesics 118
  non-opioids 84, 87
  non-steroidal anti-inflammatory drugs 84, 132–3
  opioids 71, 79, 135, 136, 178–9
Sigma agents 62, 64
Sigma (PCP) receptors 62. 63, 64
  drugs binding to 63, 86
Simple word scale describing pain 8
Site
  of epidural puncture 166–7
  of local anaesthetic action 95–6
  of operation
    pain at 32–3
    pain not at 34–5
  of pain 32–5, 103–4, 113–14
    assessment 6–7
SKF-10047 86
Skin grafts, anaesthesia for 171–3
Sleep, effects of pain in 46
Slow pain, fast pain and, differences between 23
Social conditioning and pain severity 37–8
Sodium valproate 89
Solubility (drug)(water), absorption related to 199–200
Source (site) of pain *See* Site
Spasm *See under* Muscle
Spinal cord
  anatomy relevant to nerve blockade 160–1
  dorsal horn 23–6
  neurotransmision within 29
Spinally applied opioids 136–8, 175–84
  future requirements 228
Spinal nerve block/anaesthesia 156–67
Spread *See also* Distribution
  of local analgesia with epidurals 165–6
  of spinally applied opioids 176–8
Staff/attendants/manpower/personnel
  analgesia administration and the role of 102, 103, 104–5
  effect of attitude 246
  future requirements 227

patient care, psychosocial aspects 40–2
view of pain 4–5
Stimulation of descending inhibition 69
Stress
  psychological 38, 39, 40 *See also* Anxiety, fear and distress
  surgical
    pain worsened by 34–5
    responses 46–55
Structures *See* Tissues, organs and other structures
Subarachnoid nerve block 157
Subcutaneous administration of analgesics 119, 120
  absorption following 201
  blood/plasma levels following 206
Subjective measurements of pain severity 8–14
Sublingual administration of analgesics 119, 121
  absorption following 200
Substance P 28–9, 30
Sufentanil, pharmacology 74
Sulindac, choice, factors affecting 133
Supervision of analgesics 101–3
Surgery *See* Operation
Sympathetic blockade 143
Sympathetic dystrophy 35, 246
Sympathetic efferent fibres 29
Syncope with local anaesthesia 148–9
Synergism, drug 232
Systemic analgesia *See* Analgesic drugs

Tazadolene, pharmacology 88
Teams, analgesic future requirements 227
Techniques of analgesic administration 116, 117, 119–28, 153–74, 183–4
  future requirements 227–8
Testosterone, postoperative levels 51
Thalamus 26
Thoracic epidural puncture 161–4
Tifluadom 79, 80
Time of onset of spinally applied opioid action 182

Timing
  of analgesia 115–16
    in drug trials 17–18
  of pain 7–8
Tiredness, patient, avoidance 42–3
Tissues, organs and other structures
  adjacent, damage to, with local
    anaesthesia 148
  associated with source of pain 33
  damage, pain caused by,
    mechanism 28–9
  drug levels 203, 204, 206
  irritation with local anaesthesia
    147–8
Tolerance
  opioid 71
  to pain, in drug addicts 44
Tolmetin, choice, factors affecting
  133
Topical application of analgesics *See*
  Transdermal administration of
    analgesics
Toxicity *See* Side-effects/toxicity
Transcutaneous electrical nerve
  stimulation 127–8
Transdermal/topical administration of
  analgesics 119, 120
  absorption following 200
Transmitters *See* Neurotransmitters
Treatment *See* Management
Trials, analgesic, assessment 16–19

U50488/U69593/U62066,
  pharmacology 79, 80
Unconciousness
  effect of pain during 46
  recovery from, explaining to
    patient about 41–2
Unmyelinated (C) fibres 21, 22, 23,
  24, 25
Urinary retention 180

Valproate, sodium 89
Valproic acid *See* Valproate
Value of pain 1
Vascular complications of local
  anaesthesia 146–7
Vasoconstrictors in local anaesthetics
  97, 146, 149, 151
Vasopressin, 8-arginine,
  postoperative levels 53–4
Ventilation and respiration (rate of)
  depression
    management 241
    neonatal/infantile 186–7
    opioid-assciated 178–80,
      186–7, 240, 241
  drug distribution and elimination
    affected by 215–16
  effects of pain on 49
  monitoring 43
  equipment, future requirements
    226–7
  pain severity measured from
    changes in 15
Vinblastine 100
Vincristine 100
Visual analogue scale 8–10

Water balance *See* Fluid balance
Weight, patient, and drug distribution
  and elimination 213–14
    See also Obese patients
Win-48098-6 84–5
Withdrawal, opioid, problems
  associated with 43–5
Words for pain
  pain severity measured using 8
  significance 2–3
Wound, operative, cannulation 156
  See also Incision, site of

Xorphanol, pharmacology 80–1
Xylazine, pharmacology 88